W9-ASQ-912

3 4028 00000

HARRIS COUNTY PUBLIC LIBRARY

641.563 Fam
The family style soul food
diabetes cookbook

$16.95
ocm70668773
04/22/2008

The Family Style
SOUL FOOD
Diabetes Cookbook

Roniece A. Weaver, MS, RD, LD
Rojean L. Williams, MS, RD, LD
Fabiola D. Gaines, RD, LD
Shawn Fralin, the Rakkasan Chef

◢◣® American Diabetes Association®

Cure • Care • Commitment®

Director, Book Publishing, John Fedor; *Managing Editor, Book Publishing*, Abe Ogden; *Acquisitions Editor, Consumer Books*, Robert Anthony; *Editor*, Greg Guthrie; *Production Manager*, Melissa Sprott; *Composition*, American Diabetes Association; *Cover Design*, Kathy Tresnak, Koncept, Inc.; *Cover Photography*, John Burwell, Burwell Photography; *Cover Food Styling*, Anne McLaughlin Nechkov; *Recipe Photography*, John Burwell; *Recipe Food Styling*, Claudia Burwell, Burwell Photography; *Printer*, Transcontinental Printing.

©2006 by the American Diabetes Association, Inc. All Rights Reserved. No part of this publication may be reproduced or transmitted in any form or by any means, electronic or mechanical, including duplication, recording, or any information storage and retrieval system, without the prior written permission of the American Diabetes Association.

Printed in Canada
1 3 5 7 9 10 8 6 4 2

The suggestions and information contained in this publication are generally consistent with the Clinical Practice Recommendations and other policies of the American Diabetes Association, but they do not represent the policy or position of the Association or any of its boards or committees. Reasonable steps have been taken to ensure the accuracy of the information presented. However, the American Diabetes Association cannot ensure the safety or efficacy of any product or service described in this publication. Individuals are advised to consult a physician or other appropriate health care professional before undertaking any diet or exercise program or taking any medication referred to in this publication. Professionals must use and apply their own professional judgment, experience, and training and should not rely solely on the information contained in this publication before prescribing any diet, exercise, or medication. The American Diabetes Association—its officers, directors, employees, volunteers, and members—assumes no responsibility or liability for personal or other injury, loss, or damage that may result from the suggestions or information in this publication.

⊚ The paper in this publication meets the requirements of the ANSI Standard Z39.48-1992 (permanence of paper).

ADA titles may be purchased for business or promotional use or for special sales. To purchase this book in quantities of 50 or more, or for custom editions of this book with your logo, contact Lee Romano Sequeira, Special Sales & Promotions, at the address below, or at LRomano@diabetes.org or 703-299-2046. For all other inquiries, please call 1-800-DIABETES.

American Diabetes Association
1701 North Beauregard Street
Alexandria, Virginia 22311

Library of Congress Cataloging-in-Publication Data

The family style soul food diabetes cookbook / Roniece Weaver ... [et al.].
    p. cm.
  Includes bibliographical references.
  ISBN-13: 978-1-58040-239-2 (alk. paper)
  1. Diabetes--Diet therapy--Recipes. 2. African American cookery. I. Weaver, Roniece, 1960-

  RC662.F35 2006
  641.5'6314--dc22
                            2006023448

Soul Food
Contents

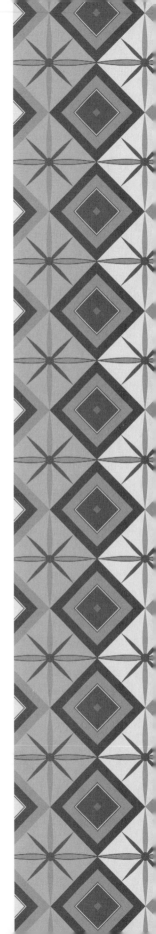

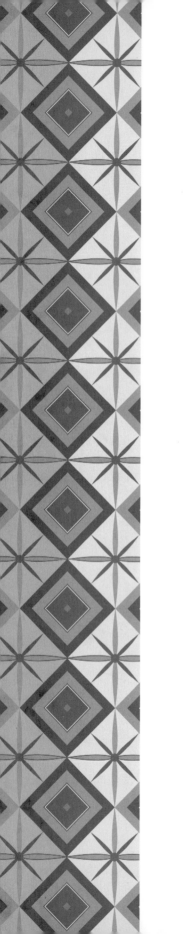

Diabetes Symptoms

◆ Frequent urination
◆ Sudden weight loss
◆ Slow-healing wound or sore
◆ Always tired
◆ Always thirsty

◆ Blurry vision
◆ Frequent infection
◆ Numb or tingling hands or feet
◆ Sexual problems

Living with Diabetes

Diabetes does not go away, but you can manage your diabetes and manage your blood sugar with these lifestyle changes.

◆ Healthy eating
◆ Exercise
◆ Medications

You can make these changes happen if you have a plan to:

◆ Practice healthy eating habits
◆ Get regular exercise (30 minutes to 1 hour a day)
◆ Take your medications at the right time
◆ Schedule regular checkups
◆ Check your feet every day
◆ Know your diabetes numbers (such as blood glucose, blood pressure, and cholesterol)

All of these things will help you manage your diabetes and still lead an active and healthy life.

Use the Soul Food Pyramid to Get Healthy

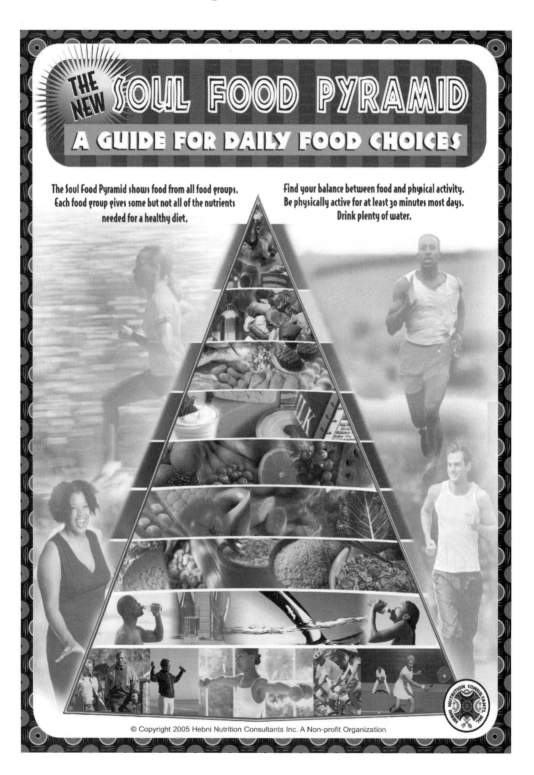

The first step to creating a healthy diet is to know what and how much you should eat. Use the Soul Food Pyramid as a guide to establish healthy eating and behaviors for your entire family.

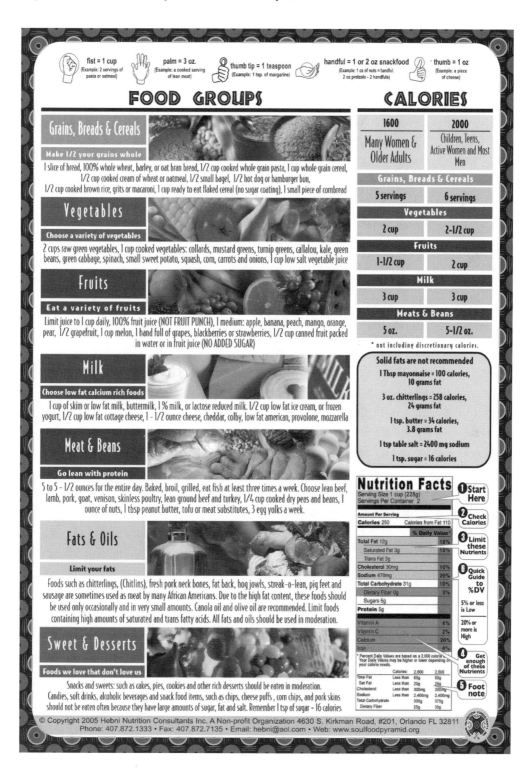

Smart Shopping = Healthy Eating

Before you begin any new habits, you must evaluate old habits that are easy to change. What most people don't realize is that by simply changing the way they shop, they can get a jumpstart on healthy eating. It's simple to start this process.

To start off, evaluate your pantry and refrigerator/freezer. What's inside? How healthy are the foods in your kitchen? If you take away the unhealthy foods in your kitchen, then you won't eat them. Replace all of those unhealthy ingredients with healthier options and you'll suddenly find that your recipes have become a part of a healthy diet. So, the first step is to eliminate or throw away the items in your pantry that are high in fat or in calories. Create a new shopping list that focuses on heart-healthy foods.

Healthy Helpings at the Grocery Store

When you're working your way through the grocery store on your next visit, start by cycling around the walls of the store before you weave through aisle after aisle. A lot of times, the freshest, healthiest foods are stored along the walls, such as fresh vegetables, breads, dairy, and meats. A lot of processed foods that can last forever are stored in the middle aisles. In the meantime, while you're doing your shopping, try to pick up these healthier versions of the foods you already buy.

• •

Breads, Cereals, Rice, and Pasta Group
◆ Breads: whole wheat, rye, or pumpernickel*
◆ Buns, dinner rolls, bagels, English muffins, and pita breads*
◆ Reduced-fat crackers: such as bread sticks, saltines, or rice crackers*
◆ Soft tortillas: corn or whole wheat
◆ Hot and cold cereals: such as oatmeal and cereal made from whole grains*
◆ Pasta: such as spaghetti or macaroni
◆ Rice: brown, wild, basmati, white, or jasmine
◆ Grains: bulgur, couscous, quinoa, barley, hominy, millet

*If you are watching your sodium intake, be sure to check the food label to find low-sodium varieties.

Fruit and Vegetable Group
◆ Fruits: any fresh, canned, dried, frozen fruit can be healthy, as long as it does not have added sugar
◆ Vegetables: any fresh, frozen, or canned vegetables can be

healthy, as long as it does not have cream or cheese sauce
◆ Fresh or frozen juices, without added sugar

*If you are watching your sodium intake, be sure to check the label to find low-sodium varieties.

Milk, Yogurt, and Cheese Group
◆ Nonfat or 1% milk
◆ Cheese with 3 grams of fat or less per serving*
◆ Low-fat or nonfat yogurt

*If you are watching your sodium intake, be sure to check the label to find low-sodium varieties.

Meat, Poultry, Fish, Dry Beans, Eggs, and Nuts Group
◆ Lean cuts of meat
◆ Beef: eye of round, top round, sirloin
◆ Pork: tenderloin, sirloin, top loin
◆ Veal: shoulder, ground veal, cutlets, sirloin
◆ Lamb: leg shank
◆ Ground beef: lean or extra lean
◆ Chicken or turkey: white or light meat (skin removed)
◆ Luncheon meats: 95–99% fat free
◆ Fish: most white meat fish is very low in fat, saturated fat, and cholesterol
◆ Tuna: light chunk meat packed in water
◆ Shellfish: shrimp, scallops, crab*
◆ Dry peas and beans: black-eyed peas, chick peas, kidney beans, lentils, navy beans, soybeans, split peas
◆ Peanut butter: reduced-fat varieties
◆ Tofu (soy beans)
◆ Eggs: egg whites or egg substitutes

*Shellfish is very high in cholesterol. Limit the amount you eat so you don't consume more than 300 milligrams of cholesterol per day.

Sweets and Snacks
◆ Low-fat cookies: animal crackers, fig bars, ginger snaps, graham crackers, vanilla or lemon wafers
◆ Angel food cake or other low-fat cakes
◆ Reduced-fat frozen yogurt, ice milk, fruit ices, sorbet, sherbet
◆ Pudding (made with nonfat milk), gelatin desserts
◆ Popcorn without butter or oil, pretzels, baked tortilla chips*

*If you are watching your sodium intake, be sure to check the label to find low-sodium varieties.

Fats and Oils
◆ Margarine: soft, light, tub varieties*
◆ Vegetable oil: canola, olive, corn, peanut, sunflower, safflower, or sesame oil

*If you are watching your sodium intake, be sure to check the label to find low-sodium varieties.

Miscellaneous/Condiments
◆ Herbs
◆ Spices
◆ Nonstick cooking spray
◆ Imitation butter (flakes or buds)
◆ Reduced-calorie or fat-free salad dressing
◆ Reduced-fat or nonfat sour cream
◆ Reduced-fat or fat-free mayonnaise
◆ Horseradish
◆ Ginger
◆ Mustard
◆ Garlic
◆ Catsup
◆ Vinegar
◆ Lemon juice
◆ Lime juice
◆ Sodium-free salt substitute
◆ Salsa
◆ Reduced-fat soups (including broths, tomato-based soups, bean soup, vegetable soup, minestrone soup)*
◆ Spaghetti sauce*

*If you are watching your sodium intake, be sure to check the label to find low-sodium varieties.

Beverages
◆ Water
◆ Sparkling water
◆ Milk: nonfat or low fat (1%)
◆ 100% fruit juice: low calorie
◆ Lemonade: low calorie
◆ Iced tea: low calorie
◆ Tea

● ●

Tips for Buying Frozen Foods

Many frozen foods and meals are high in saturated fat and cholesterol. Instead, look for frozen-food packages that say that their products are "light or lite," "lean," "reduced fat," "reduced calorie," "healthy," or "diet." These versions will be lower in saturated fat, cholesterol, calories, and/or sodium than the regular versions, but always be sure to check the food label, to be sure exactly what nutrients you'll be getting from these foods.

Tips for Buying Prepackaged, Prepared Foods

When choosing prepackaged, prepared foods, choose vegetables, pasta and grain salads, and side dishes made without high-fat mayonnaise and oil. Steer clear from dishes with high-fat meats, dressings, and other spreads (such as ground beef, creamy dressings, and cheese sauces). Fruit salad is usually available and is always a great choice.

UNDERSTANDING CARBOHYDRATES, FIBER, PROTEINS, AND FATS

It's a known fact that smart eating will help you manage your diabetes. Here are some simple facts about nutrition to keep in mind while planning your meals. Also, review the Soul Food Pyramid© for recommended servings for adults and children. Remember to look at the food labels on the packages to help determine how much of a particular nutrient will be provided by the foods you're eating.

Carbohydrate

From 45% to 65% of your calorie intake should come from foods that are carbohydrates. Scientific studies have shown that getting your carbohydrate intake to a healthier level can help reduce your triglyceride (blood fat) levels and may boost your high-density lipoproteins (HDL, or good cholesterol). Remember, carbohydrates are an essential nutrient and give energy to the brain, so you'll still need carbohydrates in your meals. The point is to choose healthier carbohydrates, such as dried beans, whole grains, fruits, and vegetables instead of sweets. You'll see that many of the recipes in this book emphasize healthy carbohydrates. Remember to strive for a higher daily intake of whole grains and fruit. Dark green vegetables are especially good for you and will fill you up.

Fiber (A Nutrient We Never Get Enough Of)

For most people, 25–30 grams of fiber per day will be enough for a healthy lifestyle. Fiber may help reduce the risks of heart disease and colon cancer and keep the digestive tract running smoothly.

Protein (A Nutrient We Get Too Much Of)

Only 10–35% of your diet should come from protein-rich foods. If more of your calories in a given day come from protein, you should think about cutting down on how much protein foods you eat per day.

Fat (A Nutrient We Get Too Much Of)

Fat sources should provide 20–35% of your daily calories, but remember that a gram of fat contains more calories than a gram of any other nutrient, such as a gram of carbohydrate, for example. Still, fat does provide some necessary nutrients and includes the healthy fats, such as corn oil, olive oil, canola oil, nuts, and seeds. Saturated fats are found in red meats, whole-diary products, butter, cheese, and some baked goods and should in general be avoided as much as possible. Trans fats, such as partially hydrogenated vegetable oil, are normally found in highly processed foods and commercially baked products; these fats should be avoided at all costs.

WHAT EXACTLY IS A SERVING?

The Nutrition Facts Label

The portion size that you are used to eating may actually be equal to two or three standard servings. Take a look at the Nutrition Facts label on the next page. Here are a few things to think about whenever you examine food you're thinking of buying.

◆ The serving size is 1 cup, but the actual package may hold 4 cups. If you eat all 4 cups, you are eating four times the serving, and you've quadrupled the amount of calories, fat, and other nutrients shown on the food label.

◆ To see how many servings a package contains, check the Servings per Container line on the Nutrition Facts label. You may be surprised to find that small containers often have more than one serving inside. Try as much as you can to stick to these amounts of servings.

◆ Learning to recognize standard serving sizes can help you judge how much you are eating. When cooking for yourself, use measuring cups and spoons to measure your usual food portions and compare them with standard serving sizes from Nutrition Facts labels. Do this for about a week. Put the measured food on a plate before you start eating. This will help you see what one standard serving of a food looks like compared with how much you normally eat.

Food Diaries

Another way to keep track of your portions is to use a food diary. Writing down when, what, how much, where, and why you eat can help you be aware of the amount of food you are eating and of the times when you tend to eat too much.

Typically, people prefer to use pencil and paper for their food diaries, and there are some professionally printed versions out there that you can purchase. However, there are online food diaries, and some are free. For those of you who feel very comfortable with computers and the Internet, you can look for these online and see what works for you. For more information about food diaries visit www.soulfood-pyramid.org.

Nutrition Facts

Serving Size 1 cup (228g)
Servings Per Container 2

Amount Per Serving

Calories 260   Calories from Fat 120

	% Daily Value*
Total Fat 13 g	20%
Saturated Fat 5g	25%
Trans Fat 2g	
Cholesterol 30 mg	10%
Sodium 660mg	28%
Total Carbohydrate 31 g	10%
Dietary Fiber 0g	0%
Sugars 5g	
Protein 5g	

Vitamin A 4%	•	Vitamin C 2%
Calcium 15%	•	Iron 4%

*Percent Daily Values are based on a 2,000 calorie diet. Your Daily Values may be higher or lower depending on your calorie needs.

	Calories:	2,000	2,500
Total Fat	Less than	65g	80g
Sat Fat	Less than	20g	25g
Cholesterol	Less than	300mg	300mg
Sodium	Less than	2,400mg	2,400mg
Total Carbohydrate		300g	375g
Dietary Fiber		25g	30g

Calories per gram:
Fat 9   •   Carbohydrate 4   •   Protein 4

• •

Online Food Diaries and How They Work

An online food diary gives you the tools you need to make good, healthy decisions about eating and exercise. Usually, an online provider will include a food diary, an exercise log, charts, reports, and body logs.

Online food diaries are easy to use. They allow you to simply search a food database and add what you've eaten to the food diary. These programs are designed to take the information that you have entered and give you suggestions about how to improve your diet or how to stay within your calorie goals. Some online diaries also will track your consumption of fat, saturated fat, carbohydrates, sugars, fiber, sodium, cholesterol, vitamin A, vitamin C, iron, calcium, and water.

• •

Portion Distortion

You've probably heard quite a bit about portions and servings lately, especially about how large they have become. The first thing to remember is that they aren't the same things.

A "portion" can be thought of as the amount of a specific food you choose to eat for a meal or snack. Portions, of course, can be bigger or smaller than the recommended serving sizes on the packaging.

A "serving" is a unit of measurement that is used to describe the recommended amount of a food in order to provide the necessary nutrients from the food groups. A serving is the amount of food listed on the Nutrition Facts panel on packaged food or the amount of food recommended in the Food Guide Pyramid and the Dietary Guidelines for Americans.

For example, 6–11 servings of whole grains are recommended daily. A single recommended serving of whole grains would be one slice of whole-wheat bread or 1/3 to 1/2 cup of brown rice or whole-wheat pasta. Don't confuse the recommendation to mean 6–11 portions, with no regard to size. So a sandwich with two slices of bread would be equal to two whole grain servings. The way to remember this is that portion sizes change, but number of servings doesn't. Keep an eye on portion size to see how the portions you are eating compare with your recommended servings.

This difference between portions and servings is important because portions in restaurants, for prepackaged foods, and in the home have become noticeably larger than they were in the past. Larger portions mean more nutrients and more calories. However, our lifestyles have a lot less activity in them than they used to, so we don't burn off the extra calories we're taking in from all of this food. Here is a healthy tip for portion control: eat your meals on a smaller plate and drink from a smaller glass.

WATCHING WHAT YOU EAT

The easiest way to watch what you're eating, especially for people with diabetes, who have to carefully watch their blood sugar levels, is to count carbohydrates. Everyone knows how to count, so this makes for a pretty simple way to watch your eating habits without getting too confused. Many people with diabetes also use exchange lists to keep track of what they're eating and to ensure that their diets are healthy. In general, though, it's best to ask your doctor to help you find a registered dietitian who can help you build a healthy eating plan. He or she may decide that you should count carbohydrates, use exchange lists, or some other method. You can find a registered dietitian in your area by visiting the American Dietetic Association's website at www.eatright.org.

How to Count Carbohydrates

As we've mentioned, it is better to have a professional help you set up a meal plan and guide you in handling your daily eating habits, but we'll briefly describe how counting carbohydrates works and how you can make changes to your diet to improve health.

• •

Carbohydrate Counting: Step by Step

Step 1: Determine your calorie level
Men: 2,000 calories
Women: 1,600 calories

Step 2: 50% of your calories must come from carbohydrates
Men: 1,000 calories
Women: 800 calories

Step 3: Divide your calories from carbohydrates by 4. (You do this because 1 gram of carbohydrate has about 4 calories.)
Men: 250 g carbohydrates
Women: 200 g carbohydrates

Step 4: Read food labels or follow a meal plan in order to consume 200 (for women) or 250 (for men) grams of carbohydrates each day.

Remember, this is a beginning step and not all of the facets of counting carbohydrates. Each person will have different dietary needs that will need to be addressed in their personal meal plan. This is why it is best to have an appointment with a registered dietitian, who can help you develop the meal plan that suits your needs.

• •

Carbohydrate Counting in Action

A Typical Daily Meal Plan (Carbohydrates Only)

Food	Serving Size	Carbohydrate (in grams)
BREAKFAST		
Grits, corn	1 1/2 cups	47.1
Toast, white	2 slices	22
Juice, all	24 ounces	75
Jelly, any	2 Tbsp	27
Pancakes	1 (3–4 inches)	36.5
TOTAL		207.6
LUNCH		
French fries	1 super size order	56.1
Triple hamburger	3 breads	42.5
Soda	24 ounces	96
Apple pie	1 large slice	30
TOTAL		224.6
DINNER		
Rice, white, long grain	1 cup	57.2
Dinner rolls	2 rolls	28
Sweet potato pie	1 large slice (1/4 pie)	54
Collard greens, frozen	1 cup	12.2
Punch	24 ounces	96
TOTAL		247.4
SNACK		
Popcorn, microwave	6 cups	22
Cookies, chocolate chip	10 cookies	62.4
Soda	24 ounces	96
TOTAL		180.4

Grand total of daily carbohydrates: **860 grams**

*This chart only shows carbohydrates consumed. Fats and proteins are not listed, but they do contribute to your total daily caloric intake. The focus of this chart is to give you an idea of what your total daily carbohydrate intake might be.

A Healthier Daily Meal Plan

Food	Serving Size	Carbohydrate (in grams)
BREAKFAST		
Grits, corn	1 cup	31.4
Toast, white	1 slice	11
Fruit cocktail, water packed	1/2 cup	10.4
TOTAL		52.8
LUNCH		
French fries	1 large	36.3
Chicken nuggets	6 pieces	16.5
Catsup	5 Tbsp	5
TOTAL		57.8
DINNER		
Sweet potato pie	1 slice (1/8 pie)	27
Collard greens, frozen	1 cup	12.2
Dinner roll	1 roll	14
TOTAL		53.2
SNACK		
Popcorn, microwave	3 cups	11
TOTAL		11
Grand total of daily carbohydrates:		**174.8 grams**

• •

100 Ways to Cut 100 Calories

Maintaining a healthy weight depends on achieving energy balance. This is accomplished by balancing the amount of energy burned and food consumed in your day. To stop weight gain, most Americans need to do just two simple things:

◆ Add 2,000 more steps each day

◆ Eat 100 fewer calories daily

Small changes in the types of foods you eat and in the portion sizes you choose will quickly add up to 100 reduced calories, or even more! By pledging to walk an extra mile (equivalent to 2,000 steps) and reduce 100 calories (equivalent to 1 tablespoon of butter) you'll see how easy it can be to achieve energy balance. Find ways to cut calories during your day with this list of ideas.

Breakfast

Give your day a healthy start with these breakfast tips:

- ◆ Select nonfat or 1% milk instead of whole milk
- ◆ Use a small glass for your juice and a small bowl for your cereal
- ◆ Savor a bowl of bananas, berries, low-fat milk, and sugar substitute
- ◆ Substitute a no-calorie sweetener for sugar in your coffee, tea, and cereal
- ◆ Choose light yogurt made with no-calorie sweetener
- ◆ Substitute no-sugar-added jelly or jam for the sugar-rich varieties
- ◆ Spread your muffin, bagel, or toast with 2 teaspoons of fat-free or light cream cheese
- ◆ Split a bagel with someone, or wrap up the other half for tomorrow's breakfast
- ◆ Use a nonstick skillet and cooking spray in place of butter or margarine to prepare your eggs
- ◆ Try turkey sausage or Canadian bacon for less fat than regular
- ◆ Fill your omelet with onions, peppers, spinach, and mushrooms instead of cheese and meat
- ◆ Lighten up your omelet, frittata, or scrambled eggs by using 4 egg whites or 1/2 cup egg substitute
- ◆ Trade regular butter for light whipped or low-calorie butter substitute.

Lunch/Dinner

Try these ideas for lighter lunches and downsized dinners:

- ◆ Put lettuce, tomato, onions, and pickles on your burger or sandwich instead of cheese
- ◆ Prepare tuna or chicken salad with a smaller amount of fat-free or light mayonnaise
- ◆ Grill your sandwich using nonstick cooking spray instead of butter
- ◆ Stuff a pita pocket with more fresh vegetables, less meat and cheese
- ◆ Pick water-packed tuna instead of tuna packed in oil
- ◆ Wrap romaine and sprouts with smoked ham or turkey in a tortilla
- ◆ Make your sandwich with light, whole-wheat bread
- ◆ Try a veggie burger

- ◆ Select soft taco size (6–8 inch) flour tortillas instead of the larger burrito size
- ◆ Substitute low-fat or fat-free sour cream in recipes
- ◆ Choose 1% cottage cheese
- ◆ Skim the fat off soups, stews, and sauces before serving
- ◆ Enjoy your salad without the croutons
- ◆ Substitute 2 tablespoons reduced-calorie salad dressing for regular
- ◆ Use diet margarine
- ◆ Trim all fat from beef, pork, and chicken (also remove the skin from chicken)
- ◆ Bake, broil, or grill chicken and fish rather than frying
- ◆ Limit meat portions to 3–4 ounces (the size of a deck of cards)
- ◆ Customize spaghetti sauce with fresh zucchini, green peppers, mushrooms, and onions
- ◆ Turn a mixed green or spinach salad into a main dish by including blueberries, diced apples, or strawberries, almonds, and grilled chicken
- ◆ Reduce your portion of cooked rice and pasta by half a cup
- ◆ Grill portabella mushrooms as a main or side dish
- ◆ Use 1 tablespoon less butter, margarine, or oil in your recipe
- ◆ Try reduced fat cheese in casseroles and appetizers
- ◆ Season steamed vegetables with fresh lemon and herbs
- ◆ Use vegetable cooking spray and nonstick cookware instead of butter, margarine, or oil when stovetop cooking
- ◆ Omit or use half the amount of butter, margarine, or oil called for in macaroni and cheese, rice, pasta, and stuffing
- ◆ Leave 3–4 bites on your plate
- ◆ Eat slowly to make your meal last and reduce your urge for second helpings.

Desserts

You don't have to eliminate desserts to cut 100 daily calories… instead, try these ideas:

- ◆ Satisfy your sweet tooth with a sliver, bite, or taste of dessert instead of a full portion
- ◆ Savor a root beer float with zero-calorie root beer, and 1 scoop of low-sugar vanilla ice cream
- ◆ Have a single-dip ice cream cone instead of several scoops in a bowl

- Choose your piece of sheet cake from the middle, where there's less icing
- Top angel food cake with berries and low-calorie whipped cream
- Freeze blended fresh fruit into a sorbet for a refreshing dessert
- Select a cupcake rather than a standard slice of cake
- Dish up low-calorie frozen yogurt or sherbet instead of ice cream
- Enjoy a dish of fresh fruit in season instead of custard or pudding
- Choose apple, peach, or blueberry over pecan or cream pie
- Follow the low fat directions when preparing brownie, cake, and cookie mixes
- Share your dessert with someone else
- Cut a half slice of cake or pie
- Substitute half or all the oil in a recipe with applesauce when baking.

Snacks

Curb your hunger with these healthy snack ideas:

- Freeze grapes or watermelon wedges for a popsicle-like treat
- Blend a smoothie out of yogurt, low-fat milk, and fresh fruit
- Choose 4 ounces of light yogurt made with no-calorie sweetener
- Manage your portions by pouring an individual serving of pretzels or chips into a bowl instead of eating from the bag
- Mix fruit in a no-sugar gelatin for a colorful snack
- Try hummus with pita wedges
- Enjoy canned fruit packed in water or its natural juice instead of heavy syrup
- Pick a small piece of fruit (apple, peach, orange) the size of a tennis ball, or eat just half of a bigger piece of fruit
- Make kabobs with fresh fruit and reduced-fat cheese
- Dip apples in low-fat caramel, celery in lite cream cheese, veggies in low-fat dressing, or fruit in a yogurt/orange juice mix
- Try fresh fruit in place of dried fruit
- Eat just 1 of the granola/snack bars in the package and share the other or save it for later
- Have 1 less handful of mixed nuts
- Satisfy your chocolate craving with by opting for 1 or 2 small "fun size" candy bars, or just a few M&Ms or Kisses
- Munch on a small bag of microwave popcorn—and don't add butter
- Eat 2 of your favorite packaged cookies instead of 3.

Beverages

Try these lower calorie thirst quenchers:

◆ Substitute diet soda for regular soda

◆ Pay attention to serving sizes, most soda cans contain 2 servings

◆ Select diet flavored iced tea

◆ Quench your thirst with bottled water instead of soda from the vending machine

◆ Opt for the small or medium drink instead of large

◆ Select nonfat (skim) or 1% milk instead of whole milk

◆ Have 1 cup of low-fat (1%) chocolate milk instead of whole milk with chocolate syrup

◆ Lighten up your favorite coffee drink by requesting nonfat milk and using half the sugar or flavored syrup

◆ Choose no-sugar-added fruit juices

◆ Replace just 8 ounces of soft drink, fruit juice, or fruit beverage with water

◆ Drink light beer—limit yourself to 1 or 2—instead of regular

◆ Request diet mixers (cola, tonic water, ginger ale)

◆ Choose light beer or wine instead of frozen or fruit-based alcoholic drinks.

Dining Out

Whether you're whipping through the drive-thru or going out for a special occasion, try these ideas for cutting calories when dining out:

◆ Limit yourself to 1 portion of bread, rolls, crackers, chips or, better yet, save your appetite for your meal

◆ Ask for a cup of soup rather than a bowl

◆ Select minestrone or other broth-based soups over cream-based soups

◆ Ask for sauce and salad dressing on the side; eat enough to enjoy the flavor, but leave most of it behind

◆ Dip your fork into the dressing, then into your salad greens

◆ Order a vinaigrette dressing rather than a mayonnaise-based dressing

◆ Ask for no croutons and cheese on your salad

◆ Substitute steamed vegetables for the potato, rice, or pasta side dish

◆ Select an appetizer as your main dish; add soup, salad, or vegetable side dish

◆ Choose a healthy option item designated by a symbol on the menu

◆ Ask for a half-portion or don't eat everything on your plate

- ◆ Use fresh lemon to season fish instead of tartar sauce
- ◆ Choose a side salad instead of fries when ordering fast food
- ◆ Skip the super-size promotions
- ◆ Select grilled chicken in place of breaded and fried.

Permission to reprint "100 Ways to Cut 100 Calories" granted by America on the Move. ©Copyright 2005, America on the Move Foundation. Visit www.americaonthemove.org or call 1-800-807-0077.

100 Ways to Add 2,000 Steps

It's not just what we eat that's important, but how we use the calories we consume. As long as you're active enough to balance the calories you eat with the calories you burn in physical activity, you can enjoy an occasional treat and still avoid weight gain.

By pledging to walk an extra mile (equivalent to 2,000 steps) and reduce 100 calories for one day you'll see how easy it is to achieve the energy balance that can stop weight gain. Small changes in your daily activity will quickly add up to 2,000 extra steps or more! Find ways to add steps at home, at work, and at play with this list of ideas.

At Home

Household chores, neighborhood walks, and errands are great opportunities for adding steps. Try these ideas for increasing your walking:

- ◆ Circle around the block once when you go outside to get your mail
- ◆ Walk around the outside aisles of the grocery store before shopping
- ◆ Drive or walk to a nearby high school and go around the track: 4 laps equals approximately 2,000 steps
- ◆ Make several trips up and down the stairs to do laundry or other household chores
- ◆ Pass by the drive-thru window and walk into the bank or restaurant
- ◆ Stroll the halls while waiting for your doctor's appointment
- ◆ Listen to music or books on tape while walking
- ◆ Invite friends or family members to join you for a walk
- ◆ Accompany your children on their walk to school
- ◆ Take your dog for a walk
- ◆ Start a walking club in your community
- ◆ Walk to a nearby store, post office, or dry cleaners to accomplish errands

- Benefit a good cause by joining a charity walk
- Walk to your place of worship for services
- Cut the grass
- Pace around your house while talking on the phone
- Buy a walking video so you can get in your steps on rainy days
- Experience the splendor of a sunrise on an early morning walk
- Spur your imagination by observing your neighbor's landscaping and gardens while you walk—incorporate ideas from your favorites in your own yard
- Walk to a friend's house for a visit
- Try "retro walking"; walking backwards distributes your weight more evenly (be sure you're in a safe area and are aware of your surroundings)
- Keep a walking journal; in addition to tracking steps, jot down how you feel after returning from a walk—enhanced energy is a great motivator
- Focus on walking distance over speed; it's better to get in more steps at a comfortable pace than to burn out quickly
- Walk on a treadmill on rainy days or when it's too dark to walk outside
- March in place while watching your favorite TV show
- Reverse your walking routine—start in the direction where you usually end
- Boost the results of your walk by using trekking poles
- Catch up on the day's events with your spouse and children on an after-dinner walk
- Sleep more soundly at night by taking a walk a few hours before you go to bed.

At Work

Adding steps to your workday can help you reduce stress and stay alert. Try these ideas:

- Go for a walk before starting your morning commute; you'll energize yourself for the day
- Exit the bus 1 or 2 stops early and walk the remainder of the way
- Walk to work if you live close enough
- Refill your coffee cup at the machine farthest from your workstation
- Visit the restroom on the far side of the building
- Hold a meeting while you go for a walk
- Avoid elevators and escalators: take the stairs instead

- Park in the far reaches of the parking lot
- Escape the stress of a difficult day by excusing yourself for a few minutes of walking
- Walk to a nearby store to buy a treat for your co-workers
- Designate 10 minutes of your lunch break for a quick walk
- Start an office walking club
- Ask co-workers to join you on a before- or after-work walk
- Walk to co-workers' desks to speak to them instead of sending an e-mail
- Create a step competition with fellow employees—see who can get the most steps in a day
- Encourage your co-workers to join you on walks during breaks or after work
- Climb the stairs or stroll the sidewalks for a few minutes at the end of your shift
- Shake off the effects of your evening commute by walking before dinner.

At Play

Whether your leisure time is specifically for physical activity or not, there are plenty of ways to add more steps. Try these ideas:

- Walk around the campus of a nearby university or college
- Window shop while you pace through a shopping mall
- Take the long route when browsing at a shopping center—don't visit the stores sequentially
- Join a water walking class; the natural resistance of the water strengthens muscles
- Tour a museum, zoo, or nature preserve
- Circle around a swap meet or craft show before selecting your purchases
- Take up photography—walk through a scenic location on a hunt for photo opportunities
- Sign up for a community 5K or 10K walking/running event
- Hike on a wilderness trail
- Vary your pace when walking; start out slowly then increase your speed, include short bursts of speed walking, then cool down with a slower pace at the end of your walk
- Strap a length of masking tape around your child's waist (sticky side out) so they can gather pretty leaves during the spring, summer, and fall
- Drive to a new walking trail and explore the different scenery

- Contact your local visitor's bureau or historical society and sign up for a walking tour
- Volunteer to walk dogs for an animal shelter
- Organize a community clean-up day and designate areas of the neighborhood for teams to walk through and remove debris as they go
- Meet a friend for lunch at a restaurant you can walk to
- Plan a picnic with friends, family, and children and go for a walk after your meal
- Seek out bargains by walking through your neighborhood looking for garage/yard sales
- Explore nature by keeping a field guide handy when walking
- Skim the newspaper for upcoming events you can walk to such as a garden tour, high school play, or a concert in the park
- Walk around the restaurant parking lot while waiting to be seated
- Drive to a neighboring community and tour its main street on foot
- Reward yourself for step accomplishments—for example, every time you reach your step goal for the day, put a dollar in a jar and save for a special reward
- Take a step aerobics class
- Spend a day at the beach and walk the shoreline
- Watch for birds while walking, especially during the fall migration
- Get lost in a corn maze (many are set up during autumn)
- Entice your kids to join you by turning a walk into a scavenger hunt
- Stroll around the field while watching your child's sporting event
- Play a round of golf but pass on the cart
- Instead of talking on the phone with a friend, meet for a walk and talk
- Walk with your kids to the local park.

Variety is the Spice of Life

Other activities can count toward your daily steps. Here are some ideas for adding "steps" through minutes spent in other physical activities:

- Sign up for a water aerobics class
- Join a beach or indoor volleyball team
- Play America's favorite pastime—baseball or softball
- Hit the tennis courts
- Dance the night away at a club
- Don't forget the household activities, such as scrubbing floors and vacuuming

- Weed, hoe, rake, and prune—gardening is an everyday way to be more active
- Paddle away calories on a raft, kayak, or canoe trip
- Tour a local trail by bike
- Try in-line skating through your neighborhood
- Take a class in judo or karate
- Swoosh down the slopes—try downhill skiing
- Snowshoe over hills and drifts in the colder months
- Ice skate at a local ice rink
- Enjoy the calm of nature while cross-country skiing on a trail
- Swim laps in a pool—vary your stroke for the best results
- Dive into a lake, river, or ocean for some summertime fun
- Join a Tai Chi or Yoga class for flexibility and relaxation
- Sign up for an aerobics session
- Water-ski over the waves
- Ride your bike to accomplish errands such as going to the library or depositing your paycheck.

Permission to reprint "100 Ways to Add 2,000 Steps" granted by America on the Move. ©Copyright 2005, America on the Move Foundation. Visit www.americaonthemove.org or call 1-800-807-0077.

The Importance of Blood Sugar Testing

Do You Know Your A1C?

If you have diabetes, your doctor has probably given you the HbA1$_c$ test. This test provides an accurate average of your blood sugar over a period of 2–3 months. The higher your glucose level, the higher the percentage.

A1C Test Result Guide

A1C (%)	5	6	7	8	9	10	11	12
Blood sugar (mg/dl)	90	135	170	205	240	275	310	345

People without diabetes have A1C values between 4 and 6%. If you have diabetes, aim for an A1C result that is less than 7%. An increase of 1% in your A1C can indicate a higher risk of developing diabetes-related complications, such as eye disease, heart disease, nerve damage, kidney damage, and stroke. Do your best to monitor your blood sugar levels every day and to track your condition.

Questions You Should Ask...

◆ How often should I have my A1C checked?
◆ What do my results mean?
◆ How will my medications improve my test results?

Low Blood Sugar

Part of living with diabetes is learning to cope with some of the problems that go along with having the disease. Hypoglycemia or low blood glucose (sugar) is one of those problems. Hypoglycemia happens from time to time to everyone who has diabetes.

Hypoglycemia, often called low blood sugar, can happen even during those times when you're doing all you can to manage your diabetes. But, although many times you can't prevent it from happening, low blood sugar can be treated before it gets worse. For this reason, it's important to know what hypoglycemia is, what symptoms of hypoglycemia are, and how to treat hypoglycemia.

Hypoglycemia and Its Symptoms

You are more likely to have low blood sugar when you:
◆ skip a meal or delay a snack
◆ do not eat enough at a meal
◆ take too much diabetes medication or insulin
◆ are more active during the day than usual.

The symptoms of hypoglycemia include:
◆ Shakiness
◆ Dizziness
◆ Sweating
◆ Hunger
◆ Headache
◆ Sudden moodiness or behavior changes, such as crying for no apparent reason
◆ Clumsy or jerky movements
◆ Seizure
◆ Difficulty paying attention, or confusion
◆ Tingling sensations around the mouth

What should you do?

If you think you have low blood sugar, it's always best to treat first and ask questions later. When in doubt, treat first.

Check your blood sugar level. If your blood sugar is less than 70 mg/dl, have one of the snacks listed below:

◆ 2 Tbsp raisins
◆ 4 oz juice
◆ 4 glucose tablets
◆ 5–6 hard candies

Recheck your blood sugar in 15 minutes. Have another snack if your blood sugar remains less than 70 mg/dl. You may need to follow-up with another snack if your next meal is more than an hour away.

A dietitian will help you learn how to prevent low blood sugar without adding unwanted calories. He or she can also help you identify symptoms, avoid low blood sugar, and carry the right snacks to treat low blood sugar.

Sick Day Guidelines

Colds, fever, nausea, vomiting, and diarrhea are some of the common illnesses that may cause special problems for people with diabetes. The following suggestions are for days when you have one of these brief illnesses. They are meant to help you manage these conditions and help speed your recovery.

◆ Eat your usual meal plan at your regular times.

◆ If you cannot eat solid foods, choose liquids or soft foods that you can tolerate.

◆ Drink plenty of fluids. If you have vomiting or diarrhea, try salty liquids, such as broth, bouillon, tomato juice, and broth-type soups.

◆ Test your blood sugar at least every 4 hours.

◆ If you have type 1 diabetes, you need to test for ketones at least every 2 hours while sick. If the test is positive for ketones, you should call your doctor.

◆ Take your temperature if you feel hot or have chills; you may have a fever.

◆ Take your pills and/or insulin, even if you are not eating as usual.

Coping With Diabetes: Self-Management is the Key!

The rules for diabetes monitoring are simple. If you have diabetes, you may feel that the burden is not worth all of the effort monitoring requires, but in the long run, self-management is very important and one of the best ways to avoid developing complications. Our health depends on being able to manage and have success. Learning to live with diabetes is not easy. There are many emotions attached with having this disease. The key is to learn how to manage and blend new management techniques into your daily lifestyle. Here are some tips to get you started:

◆ Do your best to monitor blood sugar levels every day and to track your condition.

◆ Learn to be patient.

◆ Find support.

◆ Discuss your feelings with your physician and nurse.

◆ Schedule a health visit with a registered dietitian (RD).

◆ Maintain a can-do attitude.

◆ Keep your action plan current.

◆ Encourage all family members to incorporate these new lifestyle changes into their lives , especially children. A team approach often helps people meet their goals.

Soul Food
New and Exciting

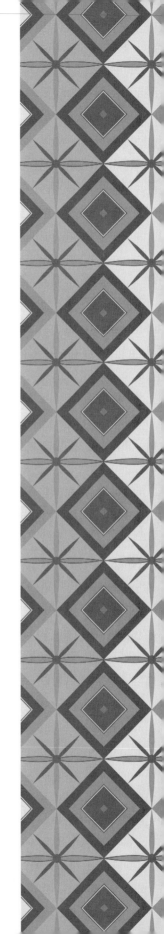

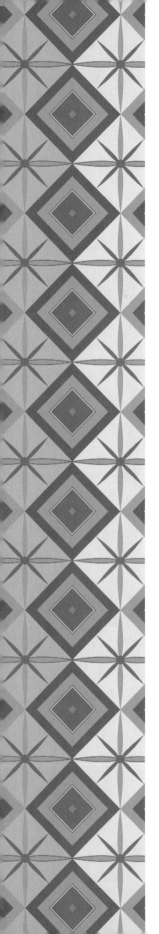

These recipes are designed to bring out the very best of soul food cooking. This means elevating the ingredients, cooking methods, and presentation of these dishes to bring the best in healthy flavors to your table.

You'll have to break away from the traditional ways of thinking how soul food should look, smell, and—most importantly—taste. The great thing is that you'll also be able to use some of those fancy kitchen gadgets more frequently. They'll no longer collect dust.

Barbeque Grilled Catfish

Preparation time: 20 min ✦ Serves 8 ✦ Serving size: 1/2 catfish

Fish

4	medium (about 1 1/2 lb each) whole farmed catfish, dressed (without head, fins, entrails, and skin)
1/2	tsp salt (1 pinch per fish)
1/2	tsp pepper (1 pinch per fish)

Barbeque sauce

1/2	tsp cumin
1	tsp paprika
1/4	tsp celery salt
2	Tbsp olive oil
1/4	cup onion, diced
2	8-oz cans tomato sauce (no salt added)
2	large whole jalapeño peppers, roasted for 20 minutes at 300°F
2	large lemons, juiced
1/2	bunch parsley, roughly chopped

1 In one dish, combine the cumin, paprika, and celery salt.

2 In a preheated saucepan, add the olive oil and the onions. Cook until browned. Once browned, sprinkle in the cumin, paprika, and celery salt, followed immediately by the tomato sauce. Then add the roasted jalapeno peppers and lemon juice. (You can remove the seeds from the roasted peppers, if you choose.) Let the sauce reduce until half remains. Add the parsley and use a hand blender to puree all of the ingredients.

3 This recipe works best if you use a fish-grilling basket to grill the fish; however, a normal grill will work just as well. Cook the fish for 30 seconds on each side. Then, using a basting brush, apply the barbeque sauce. Cook until done. Serve immediately.

Exchanges
1 Vegetable
3 Lean Meat
1/2 Fat

Calories	226	
Calories from Fat	112	
Total Fat	12	g
Saturated Fat	2.4	g
Trans Fat	0	g
Cholesterol	71	mg
Sodium	272	mg
Total Carbohydrate	7	g
Dietary Fiber	1	g
Sugars	4	g
Protein	21	g

Cornmeal-Crusted Soft Shell Crabs

Preparation time: 20 min ✦ Serves 10 ✦ Serving size: 1 crab

- 10 medium tomatoes
- 10 soft shell crabs (about 5 oz each)
- 1 cup nonfat milk
- 2/3 cup cornmeal
- 1/2 cup canola oil
- 1 tsp salt

1 Cut the tomatoes in half lengthwise. Set aside.

2 Clean the crabs. Start by cutting off the head just behind the eyes and then pull out the stomach sac. Pull back a side of the top shell to reveal the gills—they look like feathers. Pull these gills out and repeat on the other side.

3 Dip the crabs in the milk. Drain and dredge in cornmeal. Heat the canola oil in a large sauté pan. Place the crabs in the pan upside down and cook over medium heat until lightly browned. Turn over and brown the other side. Remove from pan and drain by placing on paper towels before serving. This recipe works best if served with the remoulade sauce on p. 46.

4 Arrange the sliced tomatoes on a platter. Place the soft shell crabs in the center of the platter and serve.

Exchanges
1/2 Starch
1 Vegetable
3 Lean Meat
1/2 Fat

Calories 248
   Calories from Fat 108
Total Fat .... 12 g
   Saturated Fat .... 1 g
   Trans Fat .... 0 g
Cholesterol .... 97 mg
Sodium .... 493 mg
Total Carbohydrate ..... 13 g
   Dietary Fiber .... 2 g
   Sugars .... 5 g
Protein .... 22 g

Creamy Cucumber-Dill Sauce

Preparation time: 12–15 min ✦ Serves 12 ✦ Serving size: 2 Tbsp

1	2-inch piece English cucumber (preferably diced)
1/4	red bell pepper, diced
2	Tbsp dill sprigs, chopped
1/4	tsp kosher salt
1/4	tsp white pepper
3	Tbsp lemon zest
1/2	tsp dry mustard (powdered)
1	cup plain fat-free yogurt

In a mixing bowl, combine all of the ingredients, saving the yogurt for last. Fold in the yogurt. Serve right away to prevent the sauce from becoming watery. This dish can become a creamy dressing for salad by simply adding 1 tsp of rice vinegar. The sauce can be served warm or cold.

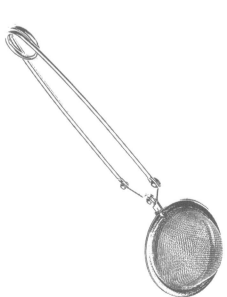

Exchanges
Free Food

Calories............................14
   Calories from Fat............. 1
Total Fat ....0 g
   Saturated Fat..................0 g
   Trans Fat ....0 g
Cholesterol ....0 mg
Sodium........................... 66 mg
Total Carbohydrate .... 2 g
   Dietary Fiber ....0 g
   Sugars ....1 g
Protein ....1 g

Fettuccine and Carrots with Lemon-Dill Sauce

Preparation time: 20 min ✦ Serves 8 ✦ Serving size: 1/8 recipe

1	cup low-fat (1%) cottage cheese
1/4	cup fat-free plain yogurt
1/3	cup shredded part-skim mozzarella cheese
2	Tbsp freshly grated Parmesan cheese
1 1/2	tsp grated lemon zest (optional)
3	medium carrots, thinly sliced
1/2	cup reduced-sodium, fat-free chicken broth
3	Tbsp lemon juice
1/4	tsp pepper, preferably white
2	Tbsp chopped scallions
1/2	cup chopped fresh dill or 1 1/2 tsp dried
1	lb fettuccine

1 Bring a large pot of water to a boil.

2 Meanwhile, in a food processor, puree the cottage cheese and yogurt until smooth. Add the mozzarella cheese, Parmesan cheese, and lemon zest (if using), and process until blended.

3 Thinly slice the carrots. In a medium saucepan, combine the chicken broth, 1 Tbsp of the lemon juice, and the pepper. Cover and bring to a boil over medium-high heat. Add the carrots, reduce the heat to low, cover, and simmer until the carrots are crisp tender, about 5 minutes.

4 Meanwhile, coarsely chop the scallions and dill, and then add to the carrots and broth. Allow this to simmer while the pasta is cooked separately.

5 Add the pasta to the boiling water and cook until al dente, about 7 minutes, or according to package directions.

6 Drain the pasta and place in a serving bowl. Add the broth and carrots, the remaining 2 Tbsp lemon juice, and the cottage cheese mixture. Toss to blend ingredients.

Exchanges
3 1/2 Starch

Calories 288	
Calories from Fat 27	
Total Fat 3	g
Saturated Fat 1.2	g
Trans Fat 0	g
Cholesterol 6	mg
Sodium 211	mg
Total Carbohydrate 50	g
Dietary Fiber 3	g
Sugars 3	g
Protein 15	g

French Toast

Preparation time: 15 min ✦ Serves 15 ✦ Serving size: 1 slice

1/4 cup Splenda® Sugar Blend for Baking
1/4 tsp cinnamon
1/2 cup pumpkin puree
1/2 cup fat-free half and half
1 cup egg substitute
1 tsp ginger
1 tsp vanilla
2 Tbsp orange juice
1/2 tsp orange zest
15 slices thick-cut, Texas-toast style white bread
3 Tbsp light, soft, tub margarine

Combine Splenda® and cinnamon in a medium bowl. Add pumpkin puree, half and half, egg substitute, ginger, vanilla, orange juice, and orange zest. Pour into a large pan. Add bread slices to pan and turn slices over to cover with mixture. Make sure the bread is covered well. Heat a skillet with the margarine. Place the bread slices into the hot skillet and brown on both sides. Serve with sugar-free syrup.

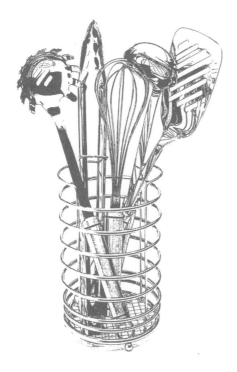

Exchanges
1 1/2 Starch
1/2 Fat

Calories..........................148
   Calories from Fat........... 29
Total Fat .... 3 g
   Saturated Fat............... 0.6 g
   Trans Fat .... 0 g
Cholesterol .... 1 mg
Sodium........................ 253 mg
Total Carbohydrate ..... 25 g
   Dietary Fiber .... 1 g
   Sugars .... 6 g
Protein .... 5 g

Freshwater Lobster Tail

Preparation time: 20 min ✦ Serves: 6 ✦ Serving size: 1 lobster tail

Broth

6	lobster shells, crushed (see instructions)
6	fresh lemon pieces (1/2 inch each)
1 1/2	cups water

Lobster

1	Tbsp lemon pepper
1/4	tsp salt
6	5-oz lobster tails, shells removed and reserved
1	tsp canola oil
2	Tbsp fresh avocados
1	whole lemon, cut into 12 wedges

1 Remove the lobster meat from the shells and set the meat aside for later. Take the shells, place them on a hard surface, and, using a pot, crush the shells (or cut them into pieces with kitchen shears). Place the shell fragments into a pot of water.

2 Add the six pieces of lemon to the shells and water. Bring to a boil and let boil until reduced by half. Strain the shells and lemon pieces from the broth and then return it to the pot. (This dish works well when served with the Yellow and White Garlic Dinner Grits, on page 54. If you choose to use this additional recipe, then about 1/3 of the broth can be used for making the roasted garlic mixture for the grits.)

3 Season the lobster meat with the lemon pepper and salt, and place it in a hot saucepan on medium-high heat with 1 tsp canola oil. Sear the lobster tails on each side. Add the avocado, lemon wedges, and half of the lobster broth. Stir.

4 Once the lobster broth begins to boil, reduce heat, and let simmer for 3–5 minutes. Serve hot. Add 1 Tbsp of pan sauce.

Exchanges
3 Very Lean Meat

Calories	94	
Calories from Fat	20	
Total Fat	2	g
Saturated Fat	0.3	g
Trans Fat	0	g
Cholesterol	126	mg
Sodium	367	mg
Total Carbohydrate	2	g
Dietary Fiber	1	g
Sugars	1	g
Protein	16	g

Fritters

Preparation time: 5 min ✦ Serves 16 ✦ Serving size: 1 fritter

2	pkg Jiffy Corn Muffin Mix (8.5 oz each)
1/2	cup egg substitute
1 1/4	cups nonfat milk
2	chili peppers, seeded and very thinly sliced
2	cups frozen corn kernels
1	cup shredded fat-free cheddar cheese
2	Tbsp canola oil

Combine the muffin mix with the egg substitute and milk to make a batter. Stir in the chili peppers, corn, and cheese. Heat a thin layer of canola oil in a nonstick large skillet, and pour a small amount of the batter into the skillet. Brown evenly on both sides for 2–3 minutes. Transfer to a paper towel–lined plate to drain. Repeat, adding and heating a little additional oil for the second batch.

Exchanges
2 Starch

Calories 137
    Calories from Fat 34
Total Fat .... 4 g
    Saturated Fat .... 1.3 g
    Trans Fat .... 0 g
Cholesterol .... 1 mg
Sodium .... 332 mg
Total Carbohydrate .... 27 g
    Dietary Fiber .... 1 g
    Sugars .... 8 g
Protein .... 6 g

Grilled Chicken Breast

Preparation time: 15 min ✦ Serves 6 ✦ Serving size: 1 breast

> 6   3-oz chicken breasts with ribs
> 2   Tbsp paprika
> 1   Tbsp ginger, powdered
> 1   dash cayenne pepper
> 2   dash cumin
> 1/4   tsp white pepper
> 1/4   tsp kosher salt
> 2   Tbsp canola oil

1 Remove the skin from chicken breast. Combine all spices and mix thoroughly. Sprinkle evenly over the face side of each breast.

2 Using your hand, pat the spices into the breast meat, so it will not fall off while cooking. Drizzle a little bit of the canola oil over each breast on both sides.

3 Grill the breasts over medium heat. When done, place them in a pan to let rest.

(As the meat rests, the drippings—or *au jus*—will settle. If you'd like, you can use the *au jus* to prepare Yellow and White Garlic Dinner Grits, on page 54.) Because this is the fatty end of the chicken, before serving, remove the ribs from the chicken breasts and slice off the lean breast meat. Serve this lean meat while hot.

Exchanges
4 Very Lean Meat
1/2 Fat

Calories	169
Calories from Fat	51
Total Fat	6 g
Saturated Fat	1 g
Trans Fat	0 g
Cholesterol	72 mg
Sodium	144 mg
Total Carbohydrate	2 g
Dietary Fiber	1 g
Sugars	1 g
Protein	27 g

Grilled Quail With Balsamic Glaze

Preparation time: 30 min ✦ Serves 12 ✦ Serving size: 1 split breast

> 12 4-oz boneless quail split breasts, skin removed
> 3 tsp rosemary, chopped
> 2 Tbsp ground pepper
> 2 Tbsp kosher salt
> 1/4 cup aged balsamic vinegar (12 years or more only)

1 Debone and remove the skin from the quail breasts. Season them with 1/4 tsp rosemary and a pinch of salt and pepper. Place the quail over medium-high heat on a grill. Cook until the quail is browned and the breast meat is medium done.

2 While the quail is cooking, place a 10-inch sauté pan over medium-low heat (this can be done on the grill). Heat the balsamic vinegar (it should be syrupy in consistency).

3 Add the cooked quail to the sauté pan with the balsamic vinegar glaze. Continue cooking; turning the breasts until they are lightly glazed and the meat is medium well. This recipe tastes best when served on a bed of 4 Tbsp black-eyed peas and 1/4 cup steamed baby spinach (not included in nutritional analysis).

Exchanges
3 Very Lean Meat

Calories......................118
   Calories from Fat..........25
Total Fat ....3 g
   Saturated Fat...............0.8 g
   Trans Fat ....0 g
Cholesterol ....53 mg
Sodium..........................531 mg
Total Carbohydrate.......1 g
   Dietary Fiber ....0 g
   Sugars ....1 g
Protein ....21 g

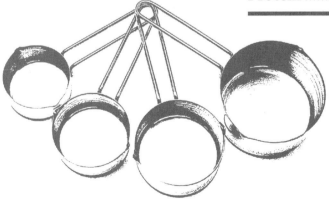

Island Shrimp

Preparation time: 20 min ✦ Serves 50 ✦ Serving size: 4 oz

16.6	lb medium-size raw whole shrimp, shelled and deveined
1/2	cup rum
2	cups vinegar
1	bottle lite soy sauce (8.3 oz)
1 2/3	cups cornstarch
1	cup canola oil
1	cup garlic, minced
2	tsp red pepper flakes
1/4	cup fresh minced ginger

1 Toss the shrimp with rum. Combine vinegar, soy sauce, and cornstarch in a bowl and mix well. Stir into shrimp and rum mixture.

2 Heat oil in a large skillet or wok over high heat and stir-fry the shrimp mixture and remaining ingredients for 5 minutes.

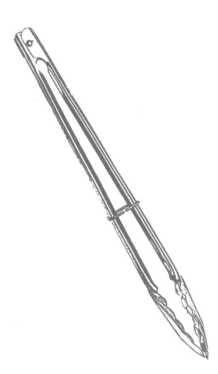

Exchanges
1/2 Starch
3 Very Lean Meat
1/2 Fat

Calories........................157
  Calories from Fat........... 49
Total Fat .... 5 g
  Saturated Fat................ 0.6 g
  Trans Fat .... 0 g
Cholesterol ....174 mg
Sodium..........................376 mg
Total Carbohydrate .... 6 g
  Dietary Fiber .... 0 g
  Sugars .... 0 g
Protein .... 19 g

Peanut Dressing or Sauce

Preparation time: 10 min ✦ Serves 10 ✦ Serving size: 2 Tbsp

    2   Tbsp peanut butter
    2   Tbsp lite soy sauce
    2   Tbsp ginger, fresh ground
    2   medium-size navel oranges, fresh squeezed
        (about 3/4 cup orange juice)
    3   Tbsp orange zest
    1   Tbsp rice vinegar
    2   tsp sesame oil
  1/4   tsp white pepper

In a mixing bowl, combine the peanut butter, soy sauce, ground ginger, and freshly squeezed orange juice. Blend thoroughly, and then add the orange zest, rice vinegar, sesame oil, and white pepper. Serve hot or cold.

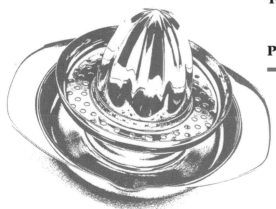

Exchanges
1 Fat

Calories 44
   Calories from Fat 24
Total Fat .... 3 g
   Saturated Fat .... 0.5 g
   Trans Fat .... 0 g
Cholesterol .... 0 mg
Sodium ....131 mg
Total Carbohydrate ...... 4 g
   Dietary Fiber .... 0 g
   Sugars .... 2 g
Protein .... 1 g

Remoulade Sauce

Preparation time: 10–15 min ✦ Serves 32 ✦ Serving size: 1 Tbsp

- 1/2 cup dill pickles
- 1/4 cup onions
- 1/4 cup capers
- 1 1/4 cups fat-free mayonnaise
- 2 Tbsp parsley, chopped
- 1 tsp anchovy paste

Chop the pickles and onions very fine. Chop the capers, if they are large, or leave whole, if small. Press the pickles and capers in a fine sieve or squeeze them out in a piece of cheesecloth, so that they don't make the sauce too liquid. Combine all ingredients in a bowl and mix well.

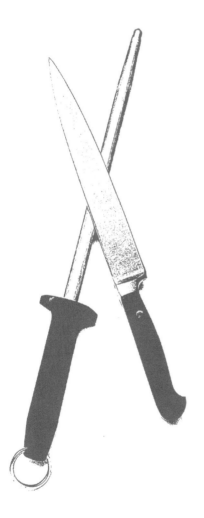

Exchanges
Free Food

Calories	8
Calories from Fat	0
Total Fat	0 g
Saturated Fat	0 g
Trans Fat	0 g
Cholesterol	0 mg
Sodium	134 mg
Total Carbohydrate	2 g
Dietary Fiber	0 g
Sugars	1 g
Protein	0 g

Rum Pork Chops

Preparation time: 15 min ✦ Serves 6 ✦ Serving size: 4 oz

- 6 pork chops (1/2-inch thick, about 4 oz each), boneless and trimmed of all fat
- 6 large sage leaves, coarsely chopped
- 6 sprigs thyme, coarsely chopped
- 1/4 tsp kosher salt
- 1/4 tsp pepper, fresh cracked
- 1 Tbsp paprika
- 1 1/2 cups rum, preferably dark and aged
- 2 Tbsp ginger, freshly minced
- 3 Tbsp garlic cloves
- 2 Tbsp Worcestershire sauce
- 1 Tbsp olive oil

1 In a shallow pan, place all of the pork chops that have been deboned and trimmed of all fat. Coarsely chop the sage and thyme. Season the pork chops with the sage, thyme, salt, pepper, and paprika.

2 In a blender, combine the rum, ginger, garlic, Worcestershire sauce, and a pinch of salt and pepper. Blend together, and then pour over the pork chops. Marinate in the refrigerator for 2 hours. Remove from the refrigerator and place the chops on a plate. Reserve the rum marinade for later. Cover the chops and let them sit for 15 minutes before cooking.

3 In a skillet, heat the olive oil. Sear the chops on a medium-high heat. Once both sides have been seared, reduce to medium heat. When the chops are medium well or 140°F internal temperature, add about 2 Tbsp of the rum marinade to the pan and shake or flip, making sure to cover each chop.

4 At this point, light the rum on fire to burn off the alcohol. If you choose not to light the rum on fire or if it doesn't catch fire, then just allow the rum to evaporate. Serve hot.

Exchanges
3 Lean Meat
1/2 Fat

Calories	199	
Calories from Fat	88	
Total Fat	10	g
Saturated Fat	3.2	g
Trans Fat	0	g
Cholesterol	51	mg
Sodium	143	mg
Total Carbohydrate	3	g
Dietary Fiber	0	g
Sugars	1	g
Protein	21	g

Smoked Fish "Mon"

Preparation time: 25 min ✦ Serves 6 ✦ Serving size: 4 oz

1	whole red snapper (3 1/2–4 lb), scaled and cleaned
1	tsp kosher salt
1	Tbsp cracked black pepper
1	medium red bell pepper, finely diced
1	medium yellow bell pepper, finely diced
1	medium sweet onion, finely diced
1/4	cup chopped cilantro
1/4	cup ginger, finely diced
1	Tbsp garlic, minced
1	medium Scotch bonnet pepper, ribbed, seeded, and diced small
1/2	cup dark rum
1/4	cup lime juice
2	Tbsp cane or dark brown sugar
1/2	cup olive oil
1	cup mesquite wood chips, soaked in water for 1 hour
	Garnish: Fresh coconut slivers

1 Make 4 or 5 deep diagonal cuts into the flesh of the fish on both sides. Season the snapper—inside and out—with the salt and black pepper.

2 In a mixing bowl, combine the red pepper, yellow pepper, onion, and cilantro; set aside.

3 Place the snapper in a large casserole dish. Stuff the cavity of the fish with the pepper-onion mixture. In a small bowl, mix the ginger, garlic, and the Scotch bonnet pepper; then rub this mixture all over the fish. Be sure to rub the cavity and the slits on both sides. *Remember to use rubber or latex gloves for this step or the Scotch bonnet pepper will burn your skin.*

4 In a separate mixing bowl, combine the rum, lime juice, sugar, and olive oil. Pour this mixture over the snapper and wrap with plastic. Refrigerate and let marinate for 2 hours before smoking. Be sure to turn the fish three times during the marinating period.

5 Set up the grill using an indirect cooking method (the coals are pushed to the sides of the grill and the fish will be cooked in the center of the grill). Sprinkle the mesquite wood chips on top of the charcoal. Place the marinated snapper in a fish basket and place the basket on the grill. Cover the grill and let the fish cook for 45 minutes to 1 hour, or until the flesh flakes and breaks away from the bone. Garnish with fresh-grated coconut.

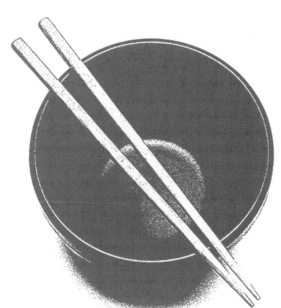

Exchanges
2 Vegetable
4 Very Lean Meat
1 Fat

Calories 246	
Calories from Fat 74	
Total Fat 8	g
Saturated Fat 1.3	g
Trans Fat 0	g
Cholesterol 55	mg
Sodium 392	mg
Total Carbohydrate 9	g
Dietary Fiber 2	g
Sugars 5	g
Protein 32	g

Spinach Fettuccine with Vegetable Ribbons

Preparation time: 15 min ✦ Serves 6 ✦ Serving size: 1/6 recipe

2	medium carrots
2	medium zucchini, unpeeled
4	scallions
1/2	lb spinach fettuccine, dry
1	cup reduced-sodium, low-fat chicken broth
2	cloves garlic, minced or crushed through a press
1	tsp oregano
1/2	tsp pepper
2	Tbsp cornstarch
1/4	cup freshly grated Parmesan cheese

1 Bring a large pan of water to a boil. Meanwhile, using a vegetable peeler, slice long ribbons off of the carrot and zucchini. Coarsely chop the scallions.

2 Add the fettuccine to the boiling water and cook until al dente, about 8–10 minutes, or according to package directions.

3 Meanwhile, in a large skillet, combine 3/4 cup of the broth with the garlic, oregano, and pepper and bring to a boil. Add the carrot and zucchini ribbons, reduce to medium-low heat, cover, and simmer until the vegetables are wilted and tender, about 3 minutes.

4 With a slotted spoon, move the carrot and zucchini ribbons to a serving bowl. Reserve the broth in the skillet. Drain the pasta and add it to the vegetable ribbons. Cover loosely to keep warm.

5 In a small bowl, combine the cornstarch and remaining 1/4 cup broth and stir to blend. Bring the broth in the skillet to a boil over medium-high heat, stir in the cornstarch mixture and the scallions, and cook. Stir frequently, until the sauce has thickened slightly, about 1 minute.

6 Add the sauce and Parmesan cheese to the pasta and vegetables and toss to coat. Serve immediately.

Exchanges
3 1/2 Starch
1 Vegetable
1/2 Fat

Calories	326	
Calories from Fat	27	
Total Fat	3	g
Saturated Fat	1	g
Trans Fat	0	g
Cholesterol	3	mg
Sodium	138	mg
Total Carbohydrate	61	g
Dietary Fiber	5	g
Sugars	4	g
Protein	13	g

Stuffed Vine-Ripe Tomatoes

Preparation time: 20 min ✦ Serves 6 ✦ Serving size: 4 oz

6	vine-ripe tomatoes (3 oz each)
2	cloves garlic
10	sprigs Italian parsley
3	large fresh sage leaves, finely chopped
1	Tbsp rice vinegar
1/4	tsp salt
1/4	tsp pepper
5	oz medium shrimp, chopped
1/2	cup diced Vidalia onion
1/2	cup diced avocado
2/3	cup romaine lettuce, chopped

1 Slice the top third of the tomatoes, keeping the tops. Remove the seeds and ribs of the tomatoes, placing them in a blender with the garlic, 5 sprigs of Italian parsley, sage, rice vinegar, salt, and pepper. Puree until smooth.

2 Place the puree in a small pot on the stove on medium-high heat. When the tomato puree begins to bubble, add the chopped shrimp, and stir thoroughly to coat all of the shrimp. Reduce to medium heat and cook for 3 minutes.

3 Take the pot off the heat and let cool. While the pot is cooling, add the diced onions. Once completely cooled, add the avocado and lettuce to the pot and mix thoroughly. Spoon the mixture into the hollowed-out tomatoes.

4 Place the tomatoes on a salad plate, with the tomato lids leaning up against the tomatoes. To make the tomatoes stand upright, shave off a little at the bottom, creating a flat bottom.

Exchanges
1 Vegetable
1 Very Lean Meat
1/2 Fat

Calories	69	
Calories from Fat	23	
Total Fat	3	g
Saturated Fat	0.4	g
Trans Fat	0	g
Cholesterol	46	mg
Sodium	157	mg
Total Carbohydrate	6	g
Dietary Fiber	2	g
Sugars	3	g
Protein	6	g

Sunny Creamy Kernel Corn

Preparation time: 5 min ✦ Serves 8 ✦ Serving size: 1/4 cup

6	ears of corn (each about 7–9 inches long)
6	Tbsp reduced-fat sour cream
1/4	tsp kosher salt
1/4	tsp white pepper
1	bunch watercress

1 Stand each of the corncobs on end and, taking a sharp knife, cut the kernels off the cob. Take half of the corn kernels and steam them for 4 minutes. Place the steamed kernels in a blender with the sour cream, salt, and pepper.

2 Puree the corn mixture until smooth. Pour the mixture into a pot. Simmer over low heat and add the remaining whole kernels. Cook until the whole kernels are soft.

3 Take 2–3 sprigs of watercress and place them on a plate. Spoon 1/4 cup of the corn over the watercress. (This recipe goes wonderfully with the Grilled Quail with Balsamic Glaze on page 43.)

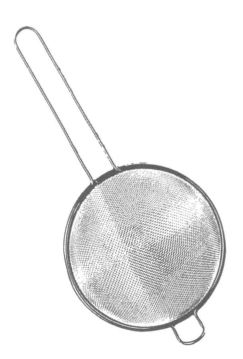

Exchanges
1 1/2 Starch

Calories	116
Calories from Fat	16
Total Fat	2 g
Saturated Fat	0.9 g
Trans Fat	0 g
Cholesterol	4 mg
Sodium	77 mg
Total Carbohydrate	25 g
Dietary Fiber	3 g
Sugars	4 g
Protein	4 g

Tuna Salmon Croquette

Preparation time: 20 min ✦ Serves 6 ✦ Serving size: 4 oz

1	large Vidalia onion, diced
12	oz canned tuna, packed in water
12	oz canned salmon
4	stalks green onions, green tips only
1	whole lemon, zested
	Juice of 1/2 lemon, fresh squeezed
1/2	large green bell pepper, diced
1/2	large yellow bell pepper, diced
4	sprigs lemon basil or sweet basil
1/2	cup bread crumbs, whole wheat
1/16	tsp salt
1/16	tsp pepper
1/2	cup egg substitute
2	Tbsp canola oil

1 In a small sauté pan, cook the Vidalia onion until translucent.

2 In a large mixing bowl, place the drained tuna and salmon meat. Fold in the cooked onions. To this croquette mixture, add the green onions, lemon zest, lemon juice, green and yellow bell peppers, lemon basil, 1/4 cup of bread crumbs, salt, pepper, and egg substitute. Mix thoroughly.

3 Form the mixture into six 4-oz patties, and then sprinkle the remaining bread crumbs over the patties. Gently press the bread crumbs into the patties. Repeat on all sides.

4 Heat the oil in a preheated sauté pan over medium-high heat. Add the patties and reduce the heat to medium. Cook the patties for 3–4 minutes on each side or until done (150°F).

Exchanges
1/2 Starch
1 Vegetable
3 Lean Meat

Calories 241
   Calories from Fat........... 80
Total Fat .... 9 g
   Saturated Fat............... 1.3 g
   Trans Fat .... 0 g
Cholesterol .... 36 mg
Sodium .... 589 mg
Total Carbohydrate ..... 13 g
   Dietary Fiber .... 2 g
   Sugars .... 3 g
Protein .... 26 g

This recipe is high in omega-3 fatty acids, which are good for your heart.

Yellow and White Garlic Dinner Grits

Preparation time: 20 min ✦ Serves 12 ✦ Serving size: 2/3 cup

    4   cups cooked yellow grits
    4   cups cooked white grits
  1/4   tsp white pepper
    6   cloves garlic, roasted
        Au jus (from chicken, shrimp, or catfish)

1 Prepare the grits according to the package instructions. This may or may not require separate cooking time.

2 While the grits are cooking, place the garlic on a nonstick cookie sheet. Roast the garlic at 325°F, until soft. Allow the garlic to cool enough to handle, so you can peel off the skin.

3 Place the peeled roasted garlic in a mixing bowl, add the *au jus* (meat juice), and whip with a whisk. Combine until you have a smooth creamy mixture.

4 Fold the garlic mixture into the cooked grits. Serve with the meat dish from which you got the *au jus*.

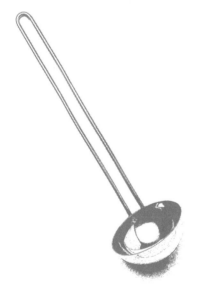

Exchanges
1 1/2 Starch

Calories............................ 98
  Calories from Fat............. 3
Total Fat .... 0 g
  Saturated Fat................... 0 g
  Trans Fat .... 0 g
Cholesterol .... 0 mg
Sodium............................. 5 mg
Total Carbohydrate ..... 21 g
  Dietary Fiber .... 1 g
  Sugars .... 0 g
Protein .... 2 g

Soul Food
Breads

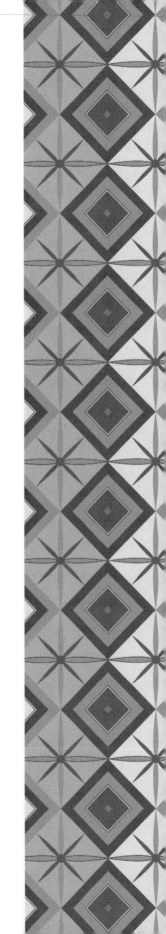

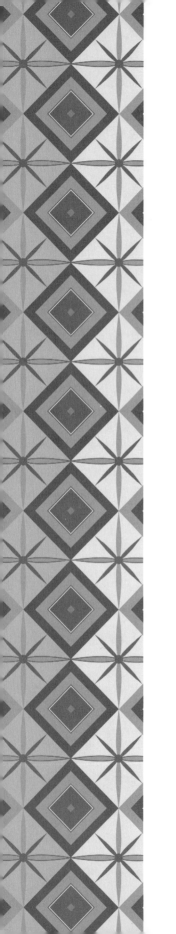

Blueberries in My Corn Bread

Preparation time: 10 min ✦ Serves 12 ✦ Serving size: 1 muffin

1   8.5-oz pkg corn muffin or corn bread mix
1   cup low-fat buttermilk
1   large egg
1   Tbsp Splenda® No Calorie Sweetener
1/2 cup dried blueberries

Preheat the oven to 400°F. Into the corn muffin mix, stir in the buttermilk, egg, and Splenda®. Fold in the blueberries. Spread evenly in a muffin pan. Bake until firm and golden brown. Serve hot.

Exchanges
1 1/2 Starch

Calories 103
  Calories from Fat...........17
Total Fat .... 2 g
  Saturated Fat .... 1 g
  Trans Fat .... 0 g
Cholesterol ....18 mg
Sodium ....187 mg
Total Carbohydrate .... 23 g
  Dietary Fiber .... 2 g
  Sugars .... 9 g
Protein .... 2 g

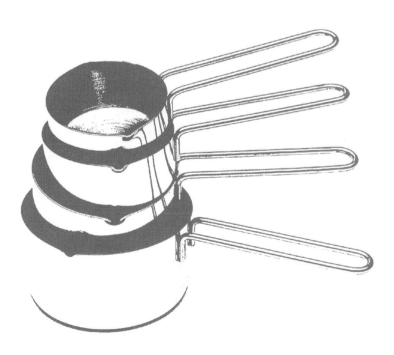

Blueberry-Lemon Muffins

Preparation time: 15 min ✦ Serves 12 ✦ Serving size: 1 muffin

1 1/2	cups all-purpose flour
1/2	cup yellow cornmeal
1/2	cup sugar
1 1/2	tsp baking powder
1/2	tsp baking soda
1/4	tsp salt
1	cup blueberries
1	cup low-fat buttermilk
3	Tbsp light stick margarine, melted
1	Tbsp grated lemon rind
1/4	cup egg substitute, lightly beaten
	Nonstick cooking spray
1	Tbsp Splenda® Sugar Blend for Baking

1 Preheat oven to 400°F.

2 Lightly spoon flour into dry measuring cups and level with a knife. Combine flour and next 5 ingredients (cornmeal through salt) in a medium bowl. Stir in blueberries. Make a well in the center of the mixture. In a separate bowl, combine the buttermilk, margarine, lemon rind, and egg substitute; stir well with a whisk. Add this to the flour mixture, and stir just until moist.

3 Spoon the batter into 12 muffin cups coated with nonstick cooking spray; sprinkle evenly with 1 Tbsp Splenda®. Bake at 400°F for 20 minutes or until a wooden toothpick inserted in the center comes out clean. Remove muffins from pans immediately; place on a wire rack. Cool and serve.

Exchanges
2 Carbohydrate

Calories	140
Calories from Fat	16
Total Fat	2 g
Saturated Fat	0.4 g
Trans Fat	0 g
Cholesterol	1 mg
Sodium	197 mg
Total Carbohydrate	28 g
Dietary Fiber	1 g
Sugars	10 g
Protein	3 g

Bran Muffins

Preparation time: 15 min ✦ Serves 40 ✦ Serving size: 1 mini muffin

1 1/2	cups wheat bran
4	cups flour
1 3/4	tsp baking soda
1/2	tsp baking powder
1	tsp salt
2 1/4	cups Splenda® Sugar Blend for Baking
1	cup raisins
1/4	cup chopped pecans
1	Tbsp cinnamon
1	Tbsp nutmeg
1	Tbsp cloves
1	cup egg substitute
2 1/2	cups canned pumpkin
3/4	cup canola oil
1	cup water
1/2	cup unsweetened apple sauce

Combine the first 11 ingredients and mix well. Add the egg substitute and the rest of the ingredients. Stir until moist. Spoon the batter into mini muffin tins, and bake at 375°F for 20 minutes.

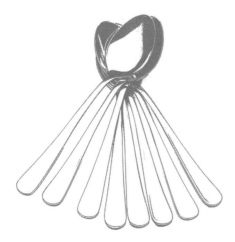

Exchanges
2 Carbohydrate
1/2 Fat

Calories........................ 158
   Calories from Fat........... 46
Total Fat .... 5 g
   Saturated Fat............... 0.4 g
   Trans Fat .... 0 g
Cholesterol .... 0 mg
Sodium..........................131 mg
Total Carbohydrate ..... 27 g
   Dietary Fiber .... 2 g
   Sugars ....14 g
Protein .... 3 g

Roberta's Buttered Sweet Potato Knot Rolls

Preparation time: 1 hour ✦ Serves 24 ✦ Serving size: 1 roll

1	pkg dry yeast (about 2 1/4 tsp)
1	cup 2% reduced-fat milk, warmed (to about 100–110°F)
3/4	cup canned sweet potatoes, mashed
3	Tbsp light stick margarine, melted
1 1/4	tsp salt
2	large egg yolks, lightly beaten
5	cups bread flour, divided
	Nonstick cooking spray

1 In a large bowl, dissolve the yeast in the milk; let stand 5 minutes. Add the sweet potatoes, 1 Tbsp margarine, salt, and egg yolks while stirring mixture with a whisk. Lightly spoon the flour into dry measuring cups and level with a knife. Add 4 1/2 cups flour to the mixture, and stir until a soft dough forms. Turn dough out onto a floured surface. Knead until smooth and elastic (about 8 minutes); add enough of remaining flour, 1 Tbsp at a time, to prevent dough from sticking to hands (dough will feel very soft and tacky).

2 Place the dough in a large bowl coated with nonstick cooking spray, turning to coat the top. Cover and let rise in a warm place (about 85°F), free from drafts, for 45 minutes or until doubled in size. (Gently press two fingers into dough. If an indentation remains, the dough has risen enough.) Punch the dough down. Cover and let rest 5 minutes.

3 Line two baking sheets with parchment paper. Divide the dough into 24 equal portions. Working with one portion at a time (keep the remaining dough covered to prevent drying), shape each portion into a 9-inch rope. Carefully shape each rope into a knot, and tuck the top end of the knot under the roll. Place the roll on a prepared pan. Repeat the procedure with the remaining dough, placing 12 rolls on each pan. Lightly coat the rolls with nonstick cooking spray; cover and let rise for 30 minutes or until doubled in size. Preheat oven to 400°F.

4 Uncover the rolls. Bake for 8 minutes at 400°F, with one pan on the bottom rack and the other on the second rack from top. Rotate pans; bake for another 7 minutes or until rolls are golden brown on top and sound hollow when tapped.

5 Remove the rolls from the pans; place on wire racks. Brush rolls with 2 Tbsp butter. Serve warm or at room temperature.

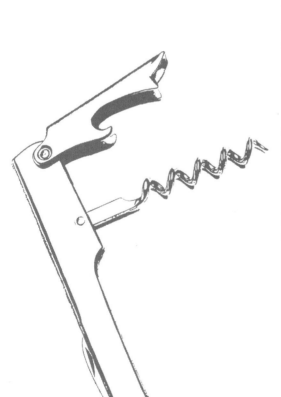

Exchanges
1 1/2 Starch

Calories	127	
Calories from Fat	16	
Total Fat	2	g
Saturated Fat	0.4	g
Trans Fat	0	g
Cholesterol	19	mg
Sodium	141	mg
Total Carbohydrate	23	g
Dietary Fiber	1	g
Sugars	2	g
Protein	4	g

Candace's Sweet Biscuits

Preparation time: 30 min ✦ Serves 8 ✦ Serving size: 1 biscuit

> 3/4 cup cooked mashed sweet potatoes
> 1/4 cup nonfat milk
> 4 Tbsp light stick margarine
> 1 1/2 cups all-purpose flour
> 4 tsp baking powder
> 2 Tbsp Splenda® No Calorie Sweetener
> 1/2 tsp salt

1 In a large bowl, mix the sweet potatoes, nonfat milk, and margarine. In a separate bowl, sift the flour, baking powder, Splenda®, and salt.

2 Combine both mixtures to make a soft dough. Turn the dough out onto a floured board and toss until smooth.

3 Roll out until the dough is 1/2 inch thick. Cut the dough with a biscuit cutter or small glass. Place on a greased pan and bake at 450°F for 15 minutes.

Exchanges
2 Starch

Calories 148
 Calories from Fat 25
Total Fat .... 3 g
 Saturated Fat .... 0.6 g
 Trans Fat .... 0 g
Cholesterol .... 0 mg
Sodium ....372 mg
Total Carbohydrate ..... 27 g
 Dietary Fiber .... 1 g
 Sugars .... 3 g
Protein .... 3 g

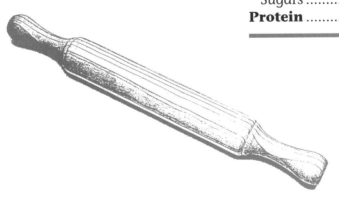

Carolyn's Texas-Style Corn Bread Dressing

Preparation time: 30 min ✦ Serves 30 ✦ Serving size: 1/3 cup

Corn bread

Nonstick cooking spray

1	cup self-rising cornmeal
1	cup self-rising flour
3/4	cup low-fat buttermilk
1/2	cup egg substitute
2	Tbsp olive oil

Dressing

2	cups onion, chopped
1 1/2	cups celery, chopped
1 1/2	cups bell pepper, chopped
3/4	cup egg substitute
1	10.75-oz can 98% fat-free cream of celery soup
4	Tbsp light stick margarine
1 1/2	tsp sage
1	tsp thyme
1/2	tsp black pepper
1	16-oz bag of herb dressing mix
4	10.5-oz cans low-fat, reduced-sodium chicken broth

Water (for moisture, if necessary)

1 Preheat the oven to 400°F. Grease muffin pans with nonstick cooking spray. Mix all of the corn bread ingredients together in one bowl. Batter should be slightly lumpy. Bake for about 20–25 minutes and set aside to cool.

2 In a heated skillet, sauté the onions, celery, and bell pepper. Cook until tender and set aside.

3 In a very large mixing bowl, combine all of the cooked vegetables and all other ingredients, including the cooked corn bread. After mixing, if the dressing is too dry, continue to add 1 can broth or water until dressing is the consistency of cooked oatmeal. Add additional spices (more sage or pepper) to taste. Bake in a preheated oven at 350°F for 1 hour or until firm.

Exchanges
1 1/2 Starch
1/2 Fat

Calories	130	
Calories from Fat	21	
Total Fat	2	g
Saturated Fat	0.5	g
Trans Fat	0	g
Cholesterol	1	mg
Sodium	450	mg
Total Carbohydrate	21	g
Dietary Fiber	2	g
Sugars	2	g
Protein	4	g

Cheese and Chive Bread

Preparation time: 20 min ✦ Serves 12 ✦ Serving size: 1 slice

Nonstick cooking spray
1 1/2 cups self-rising flour
1/4 tsp salt
1 tsp mustard powder
1 cup grated reduced-fat mild cheddar cheese
1/2 Tbsp Parmesan cheese, freshly grated
1/4 cup fresh chives, chopped
1 egg white or egg substitute
2 Tbsp light, soft, tub margarine, melted
2/3 cup low-fat milk

1 Grease a 9-inch square cake pan with nonstick cooking spray and line the bottom with baking parchment.

2 Sift the flour, salt, and mustard powder into a large mixing bowl.

3 Reserve 3 Tbsp of the grated cheddar cheese and stir the remainder into the flour mixture. Add the Parmesan cheese and chopped fresh chives and mix to combine.

4 Add the beaten egg white, melted margarine, and milk to the dry ingredients. Stir the mixture thoroughly to combine.

5 Transfer the mixture to the prepared cake pan and spread it evenly with a knife. Sprinkle the reserved grated cheese on top.

6 Bake in a preheated oven at 375°F for 30 minutes.

7 Remove from the oven and let the bread cool slightly in the pan, then transfer to a wire rack to cool completely. Cut into triangles to serve.

Exchanges
1 Starch
1/2 Fat

Calories 98
Calories from Fat 29
Total Fat .... 3 g
Saturated Fat .... 1.4 g
Trans Fat .... 0 g
Cholesterol .... 8 mg
Sodium .... 356 mg
Total Carbohydrate ..... 13 g
Dietary Fiber .... 0 g
Sugars .... 1 g
Protein .... 5 g

Cranberry Muffins

Preparation time: 20 min ✦ Serves 12 ✦ Serving size: 1 muffin

2	tsp melted light, soft, tub margarine, for greasing
1 1/4	cups all-purpose flour
2	tsp baking powder
1/2	tsp salt
3	Tbsp superfine sugar
4	Tbsp light, soft, tub margarine, melted
1/2	cup egg substitute
3/4	cup low-fat milk
1	cup fresh cranberries
1/4	cup freshly grated reduced-fat Parmesan cheese

1 Lightly grease a 12-cup muffin pan with 2 tsp margarine. Sift the flour, baking powder, and salt into a mixing bowl. Stir in the superfine sugar.

2 In a separated bowl, mix the 4 Tbsp melted margarine, egg substitute, and milk together. Pour this mixture into the bowl of dry ingredients. Mix both lightly together until all of the ingredients are evenly combined. Finally, stir in the fresh cranberries.

3 Divide the cake batter between the prepared muffin pans. Sprinkle the grated Parmesan cheese over the top of each muffin.

4 Bake in a preheated oven at 400°F for about 20 minutes or until the muffins have risen and are a golden brown color.

5 Remove the muffins from the oven and let cool a little in the pans, and then carefully transfer onto a wire rack. Let them cool completely before serving.

Exchanges
1 Starch
1/2 Fat

Calories	103	
Calories from Fat	26	
Total Fat	3	g
Saturated Fat	0.8	g
Trans Fat	0	g
Cholesterol	2	mg
Sodium	229	mg
Total Carbohydrate	15	g
Dietary Fiber	1	g
Sugars	5	g
Protein	4	g

Easy Pancakes

Preparation time: 15 min ✦ Serves 8 ✦ Serving size: 2 pancakes

> 2 cups all-purpose flour
> 1 cup egg substitute
> 1 1/2 cups nonfat milk
> 1 Tbsp canola oil
> 1 Tbsp baking powder

Mix all of the ingredients in a bowl. Be sure not to overmix; for a tender pancake, the mix should have some lumps. Place in a hot skillet and cook until golden brown.

Exchanges
2 Starch

Calories.........................160
   Calories from Fat............18
Total Fat .... 2 g
   Saturated Fat............... 0.2 g
   Trans Fat .... 0 g
Cholesterol .... 1 mg
Sodium...........................214 mg
Total Carbohydrate ..... 27 g
   Dietary Fiber .... 1 g
   Sugars .... 3 g
Protein .... 8 g

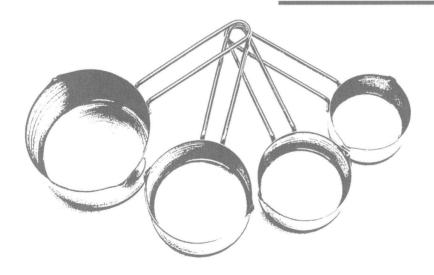

Extra Oaty Oatmeal

Preparation time: 10 min ✦ Serves 6 ✦ Serving size: 1/2 cup

- 2 cups rolled oats
- 2 Tbsp oat bran
- 1/2 cup nonfat milk
- 4 Tbsp raisins, chopped dates, or dried figs
- 1 banana, sliced
- 1 Tbsp honey or sugar-free maple syrup
- 1 tsp slivered almonds

Cook the oats, bran, and milk in a microwave for 4 minutes or on a stovetop over medium heat for 5 minutes. Transfer the mixture to a bowl and stir in the raisins or other fruit. Add the sliced banana. Add extra milk if the oatmeal is too thick. Spoon the honey or sugar-free maple syrup over the oatmeal. Lightly sprinkle with almonds and or serve with your favorite nuts.

Exchanges
1 Starch
1 Fruit
1/2 Fat-Free Milk

Calories 195
    Calories from Fat 20
Total Fat .... 2 g
    Saturated Fat .... 0.5 g
    Trans Fat .... 0 g
Cholesterol .... 2 mg
Sodium .... 47 mg
Total Carbohydrate ...... 37 g
    Dietary Fiber .... 4 g
    Sugars .... 15 g
Protein .... 9 g

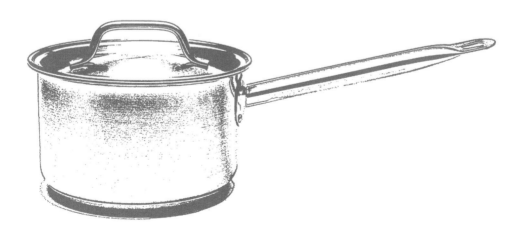

Fluffy Hotcakes

Preparation time: 15 min ✦ Serves 12 ✦ Serving size: 2 pancakes

>   3 egg whites
>   3 Tbsp light stick margarine, melted
>   1 Tbsp Splenda® Sugar Blend for Baking
> 1 1/2 cups flour
>   3/4 tsp baking soda
>   1 tsp baking powder
>   1/4 tsp salt
> 1 2/3 cups buttermilk

Beat the egg whites with a mixer at medium speed. Add the melted margarine and Splenda®. In a separate bowl, sift together the flour, baking soda, and baking powder. Beat these into the egg whites, margarine, and Splenda® mixture, while adding the buttermilk. Bake on a hot griddle or waffle iron.

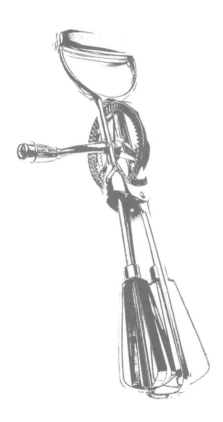

Exchanges
1 Starch

Calories 92
   Calories from Fat 15
Total Fat .... 2 g
   Saturated Fat .... 0.4 g
   Trans Fat .... 0 g
Cholesterol .... 1 mg
Sodium .... 226 mg
Total Carbohydrate ..... 15 g
   Dietary Fiber .... 0 g
   Sugars .... 3 g
Protein .... 4 g

Gold Grits

Preparation time: 20 min ✦ Serves 8 ✦ Serving size: 1/3 cup

    2 cups sweet potatoes, drained
    4 cups water
    1 cup grits
    1 tsp garlic, minced
  1/2 tsp salt
  1/2 cup light, stick margarine
    1 Tbsp Worcestershire sauce
    4 egg whites
      Nonstick cooking spray

1 In a blender, puree the sweet potatoes.

2 In a large saucepan, boil the water and add the grits, garlic, and salt. Reduce heat, stir, and cover. Cook over low heat for 15 minutes, stirring often, until the grits become thick. Add the margarine, pureed sweet potatoes, and Worcestershire sauce.

3 In a large bowl, beat the egg whites until stiff. Fold the egg whites into the sweet potato mixture. Spray a soufflé dish with nonstick cooking spray. Pour mixture into prepared dish and bake at 350°F for 40 minutes.

Exchanges
2 Starch
1/2 Fat

Calories 171
   Calories from Fat........... 48
Total Fat .... 5 g
   Saturated Fat.................. 1 g
   Trans Fat .... 0 g
Cholesterol .... 0 mg
Sodium........................301 mg
Total Carbohydrate ..... 26 g
   Dietary Fiber .... 2 g
   Sugars .... 8 g
Protein .... 4 g

Lemon Pancakes with Strawberry Topping

Preparation time: 15 min ✦ Serves 6 ✦ Serving size: 2 pancakes

Pancakes
1	cup egg substitute
3/4	cup low-fat ricotta cheese
1/4	tsp cream of tartar
1/3	cup all-purpose flour
3	Tbsp light, soft, tub margarine
2	Tbsp Splenda® No Calorie Sweetener
1	Tbsp grated lemon rind
1/8	tsp salt

Topping
Fresh sliced strawberries
Sugar-free strawberry syrup

Beat the pancake ingredients at medium speed with an electric mixer until smooth. Pour about 1/4 cup of batter for each pancake onto a hot, lightly greased griddle. Cook until the tops are covered with bubbles and the edges looked cooked; then turn and cook the other side. Serve with fresh strawberries and warm sugar-free strawberry syrup on top.

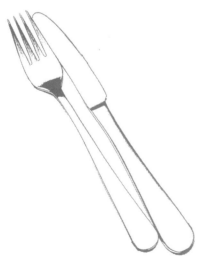

Exchanges
1/2 Starch
1 Lean Meat

Calories 98
   Calories from Fat 34
Total Fat .... 4 g
   Saturated Fat .... 1.2 g
   Trans Fat .... 0 g
Cholesterol .... 10 mg
Sodium .... 248 mg
Total Carbohydrate .... 8 g
   Dietary Fiber .... 0 g
   Sugars .... 2 g
Protein .... 8 g

Multigrain Cereal

Preparation time: 15 min ✦ Serves 24 ✦ Serving size: 1/3 cup

1/2	cup sugar-free maple syrup
1/3	cup honey
3	Tbsp canola oil
1 1/2	Tbsp vanilla extract
4 1/2	cups regular oats
1	cup uncooked quick-cooking barley
3/4	cup chopped walnuts or pecans
1/2	cup wheat germ
1/4	cup flax seed
1	tsp ground cinnamon
1/4	tsp ground nutmeg
	Nonstick cooking spray
1	7-oz pkg dried mixed fruit, chopped

Preheat the oven to 325°F. Combine the maple syrup, honey, canola oil, and vanilla extract, stirring with a whisk. Combine the oats, barley, walnuts (or pecans), wheat germ, flax seed, cinnamon, and nutmeg in a large bowl. Add the syrup mixture and stir well to coat. Spread this oat mixture evenly onto a jelly-roll pan coated with nonstick cooking spray. Bake at 325°F for 30 minutes or until browned, stirring every 10 minutes. Stir in the dried fruit. Cool completely. Store in an airtight container for up to 5 days. Serve with yogurt.

Exchanges
1 1/2 Starch
1/2 Fruit
1 Fat

Calories 183
　Calories from Fat 55
Total Fat .... 6 g
　Saturated Fat .... 0.7 g
　Trans Fat .... 0 g
Cholesterol .... 0 mg
Sodium .... 18 mg
Total Carbohydrate ..... 28 g
　Dietary Fiber .... 5 g
　Sugars .... 8 g
Protein .... 5 g

Oatmeal Bread

Preparation time: 20 min ✦ Serves 10 ✦ Serving size: 1 slice

       Nonstick cooking spray
1   cup all-purpose flour
1   cup quick-cooking rolled oats
1 1/2 tsp baking powder
1   tsp baking soda
1/4   tsp salt
1/2   cup raisins
1   tsp lemon zest
1/2   tsp cinnamon
1/4   tsp nutmeg
1/2   cup egg substitute
2   Tbsp molasses
1   cup low-fat buttermilk
2   Tbsp canola oil

1 Using a nonstick cooking spray, coat a 9 × 5-inch loaf pan and set it aside. In a bowl, combine the flour, oats, baking powder, baking soda, salt, raisins, lemon zest, cinnamon, and nutmeg. Set aside 1 Tbsp of this mixture.

2 In another bowl, combine the egg substitute, molasses, buttermilk, and oil. Stir this into the dry ingredients and blend well.

3 Spoon the batter into the prepared pan, sprinkle 1 Tbsp dry oats on top of the batter, and bake in a 350°F oven for approximately 50 minutes.

Exchanges
1 Starch
1/2 Fruit
1 Fat

Calories 152		
Calories from Fat........... 33		
Total Fat 4	g
Saturated Fat............... 0.4	g
Trans Fat 0	g
Cholesterol 1	mg
Sodium 290	mg
Total Carbohydrate 25	g
Dietary Fiber 2	g
Sugars 9	g
Protein 5	g

Orzo Pasta

Preparation time: 15 min ✦ Serves 10 ✦ Serving size: 2/3 cup

1	small onion, chopped
2	Tbsp olive oil
1 3/4	cups orzo pasta
1/2	cup shredded carrots
1	14-oz can lower-sodium beef bouillon
1 1/4	cup water
1	7-oz can mushrooms, undrained
1	Tbsp Worcestershire sauce
1/2	tsp salt
1/2	tsp soy sauce

In a large skillet, sauté the onion in olive oil until tender. Add the remaining ingredients, and bring to a boil. Reduce heat and simmer for 25 minutes, until the pasta is tender and the liquid is absorbed.

Exchanges
2 Starch

Calories........................157
   Calories from Fat........... 30
Total Fat .... 3 g
   Saturated Fat............... 0.5 g
   Trans Fat .... 0 g
Cholesterol .... 0 mg
Sodium........................ 293 mg
Total Carbohydrate ..... 26 g
   Dietary Fiber .... 2 g
   Sugars .... 4 g
Protein .... 5 g

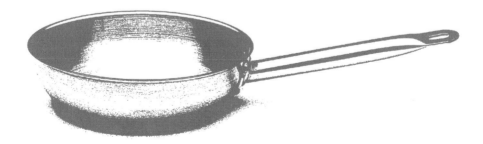

Rainbow Rice

Preparation time: 15 min ✦ Serves 10 ✦ Serving size: 3/4 cup

5	cups water
2	cups brown rice
1	tsp cinnamon
3/4	tsp nutmeg
3/4	cup raisins
1/3	tsp salt
1/2	cup dried apricots or cranberries, chopped
3	Tbsp light, stick margarine
1/4	cup pecans
2	Tbsp Splenda® Sugar Blend for Baking

Combine water and next six ingredients. Bring to a boil. Stir and reduce heat. Cover and simmer for 45 minutes. Melt the margarine in a skillet. Add pecans and sauté until brown. Sprinkle with Splenda®. Pour over rice and serve.

Exchanges
2 Starch
1 Fruit
1/2 Fat

Calories 231
   Calories from Fat.......... 43
Total Fat .... 5 g
   Saturated Fat............... 0.7 g
   Trans Fat .... 0 g
Cholesterol .... 0 mg
Sodium..........................107 mg
Total Carbohydrate ..... 44 g
   Dietary Fiber .... 4 g
   Sugars .... 13 g
Protein .... 4 g

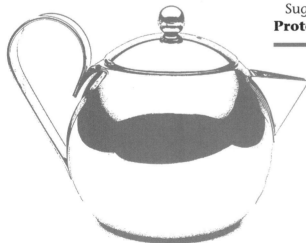

Home Fries

Preparation time: 25 min ✦ Serves 16 ✦ Serving size: 1/2 cup

- 8 large potatoes, unpeeled
- 2 Tbsp light butter
- 1 medium onion, diced
- 3 green onions, chopped
- 1/4 tsp salt
- 1/4 tsp garlic powder
- 1/4 tsp black pepper

Cook the potatoes in boiling water in a large stock pot, until slightly tender. Remove, drain water, and dice potatoes into cubes. In a large skillet, heat the butter; then sauté the onion and green onions. Add potatoes to the skillet. Season with salt, garlic powder, and black pepper. Serve hot.

Exchanges
1 1/2 Starch

Calories	104
Calories from Fat	8
Total Fat	1 g
Saturated Fat	0.5 g
Trans Fat	0 g
Cholesterol	2 mg
Sodium	53 mg
Total Carbohydrate	23 g
Dietary Fiber	2 g
Sugars	2 g
Protein	2 g

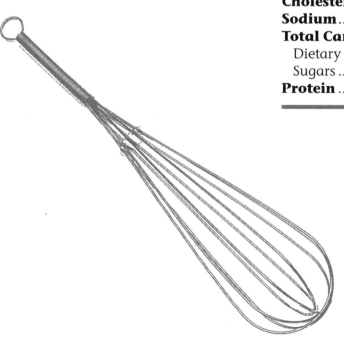

Sweet Potato Pancakes

Preparation time: 15 min ✦ Serves 12 ✦ Serving size: 2 pancakes

2	cups flour
1	Tbsp + 1 tsp baking powder
1	tsp salt
2	Tbsp Splenda® Sugar Blend for Baking
1	tsp cinnamon
1/2	cup egg substitute
1 1/2	cups reduced-fat milk
1	cup mashed sweet potatoes
8	Tbsp light, stick margarine, melted
3	egg whites, whipped

1 Combine the flour, baking powder, salt, Splenda®, and cinnamon. Make a well in the center of the dry ingredients. In a separate bowl, mix the egg substitute, milk, sweet potatoes, and margarine. Add to flour mixture and stir until ingredients are moist.

2 Beat the egg whites until stiff peaks are formed. Fold into pancake batter. Pour 1/4 cup onto a hot griddle and flip when pancakes bubble up.

Exchanges
2 Starch
1/2 Fat

Calories	169
Calories from Fat	35
Total Fat	4 g
Saturated Fat	0.9 g
Trans Fat	0 g
Cholesterol	2 mg
Sodium	417 mg
Total Carbohydrate	27 g
Dietary Fiber	1 g
Sugars	6 g
Protein	6 g

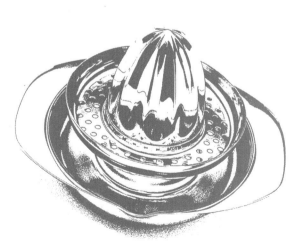

Sweet Potato Pudding

Preparation time: 25 min ✦ Serves 6 ✦ Serving size: 1/2 cup

Nonstick cooking spray
2 cups grated raw sweet potatoes
1 cup reduced-fat milk
1/2 cup Splenda® Sugar Blend for Baking
1/2 cup egg substitute
2 Tbsp light, stick margarine
1 tsp cinnamon
1/2 tsp nutmeg
1/4 tsp salt

Heat oven to 350°F. Spray a 1 1/2-quart casserole with nonstick cooking spray. Mix all of the ingredients in a large bowl. Pour mixture into the casserole dish. Bake for 1 hour or until center is firm. Serve warm.

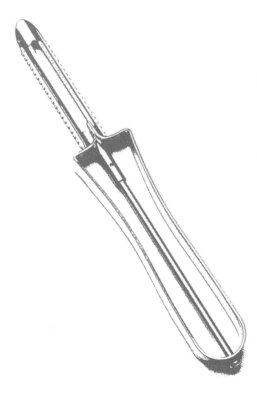

Exchanges
2 Carbohydrate

Calories 148
Calories from Fat........... 20
Total Fat .... 2 g
Saturated Fat............... 0.7 g
Trans Fat .... 0 g
Cholesterol .... 2 mg
Sodium ....185 mg
Total Carbohydrate ..... 28 g
Dietary Fiber .... 1 g
Sugars .... 20 g
Protein .... 4 g

Whole-Wheat Drop Biscuits

Preparation time: 20 min ✦ Serves 12 ✦ Serving size: 1 biscuit

- 1 cup whole-wheat flour
- 1 cup all-purpose flour
- 1/4 cup canola oil
- 1 tsp Splenda® No Calorie Sweetener
- 1/4 tsp salt
- 1 Tbsp baking powder
- 1 tsp lemon juice
- 1 cup nonfat milk
- Nonstick cooking spray

1 Preheat oven to 475°F.

2 Mix the flours, oil, Splenda®, salt, and baking powder. Pour in the lemon juice and milk and mix until all ingredients are combined. Spray baking sheet with nonstick cooking spray. Using a tablespoon, drop the biscuit dough onto baking sheet.

3 Bake for approximately 8 minutes.

Exchanges
1 Starch
1 Fat

Calories.........................121
   Calories from Fat........... 45
Total Fat .... 5 g
   Saturated Fat............... 0.4 g
   Trans Fat .... 0 g
Cholesterol .... 0 mg
Sodium..........................149 mg
Total Carbohydrate ......17 g
   Dietary Fiber .... 2 g
   Sugars .... 1 g
Protein .... 3 g

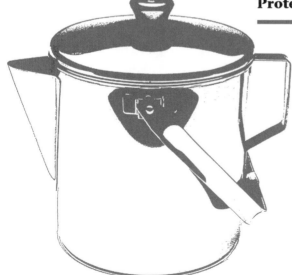

Wild Rice with Pistachios and Dried Cranberries

Preparation time: 15 min ✦ Serves 9 ✦ Serving size: 1/2 cup

- 2 cups chicken broth
- 1 cup wild rice
- 1 tsp fresh thyme
- 1/2 tsp salt
- 1 tsp black or white pepper
- 1 cup dried cranberries
- 1/3 cup chopped pistachio

Heat the broth, and add the wild rice, thyme, salt, and pepper. Add dried cranberries and pistachios after the rice is completely done. Stir well. Cranberries will rehydrate from the heat. Serve hot.

Exchanges
1 Starch
1/2 Fruit
1/2 Fat

Calories..........................119
   Calories from Fat........... 24
Total Fat .... 3 g
   Saturated Fat............... 0.3 g
   Trans Fat .... 0 g
Cholesterol .... 0 mg
Sodium........................ 350 mg
Total Carbohydrate ..... 22 g
   Dietary Fiber .... 2 g
   Sugars .... 10 g
Protein .... 3 g

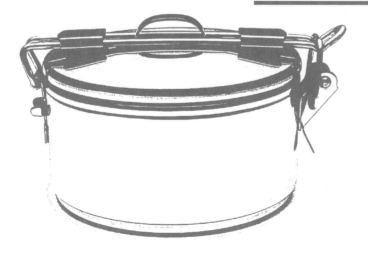

Soul Food
Vegetables

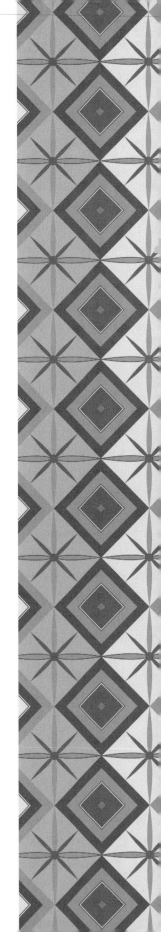

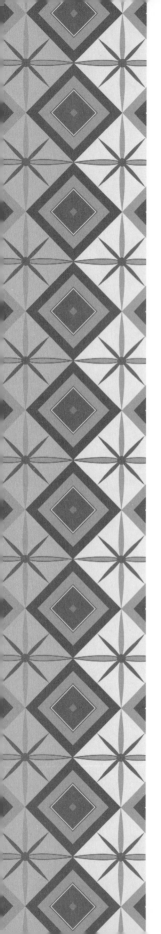

All-Mixed-Up Tofu (Stir-Fry)

Preparation time: 13 min ✦ Servings: 6 ✦ Serving size: 8 oz

1/8	tsp	cayenne pepper
2 1/2	tsp	ground cumin
2	tsp	garam marsala
1 1/2	Tbsp	paprika
2	tsp	powdered ginger or fresh grated ginger
2	lb	firm or extra-firm tofu, diced or sliced into strips like French fries
2	Tbsp	canola oil
2	cups	green beans, halved
1	cup	green bell pepper, sliced
1	cup	yellow bell pepper, sliced
1	cup	spring onions, sliced
2	Tbsp	garlic, chopped and crushed
2	cups	brown button mushrooms, halved or quartered
2	cups	zucchini, sliced
1/2	cup	pine nuts (*optional*)
1	tsp	kosher salt
1 1/2	tsp	white pepper
1	Tbsp	thyme
1	Tbsp	sage
1 1/2	Tbsp	lime juice
2	tsp	clear honey (*optional*)
2 1/2	Tbsp	rice vinegar

1 Mix the cayenne, cumin, garam marsala, paprika, and ginger in a ramekin, and then season the firm tofu. Panfry the tofu in a dab of canola oil over medium-high heat, just until they brown slightly. Remove from skillet or wok and set aside. You will add the tofu to the stir-fried vegetables just as you finish cooking them. *Remember, stir-frying is a fast high-heat cooking process. So no walking away from the stove.*

2 In the hot pan, add the green beans, bell peppers, onions, garlic, mushrooms, zucchini, and half of the pine nuts. As you stir the vegetables, add the salt, pepper, thyme, sage, and lime juice. Then add the honey, tofu, and rice vinegar. Stir several times before plating. Garnish each plate with the remaining pine nuts.

Note: If you don't have all of the ingredients, then substitute with your favorite vegetables. You can also add sesame seeds to the dish along with bean sprouts. Make this dish your own!

Exchanges
3 Vegetable
2 Medium-Fat Meat

Calories...................... 208
   Calories from Fat..........106
Total Fat .... 12 g
   Saturated Fat............... 1.8 g
   Trans Fat .... 0 g
Cholesterol .... 0 mg
Sodium..........................351 mg
Total Carbohydrate ......16 g
   Dietary Fiber .... 5 g
   Sugars .... 5 g
Protein ....16 g

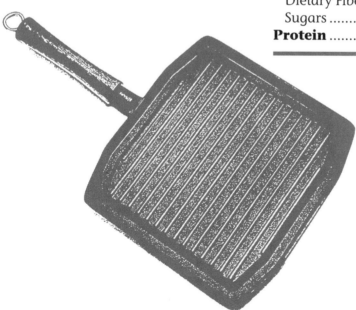

Cliff and Jennifer's Baked Beans

Preparation time: 10 min ✦ Serves 15 ✦ Serving size: 4 oz

2 bags (15 oz each) frozen onion
2 bags (15 oz each) frozen bell pepper
2 bags (15 oz each) frozen celery
2 Tbsp olive oil
1 large can (55 oz) vegetarian baked beans
3/4 cup Splenda® Brown Sugar Blend
1/4 cup water
1/4 tsp cumin
1/2 tsp cloves

1 Preheat the oven to 300°F.

2 Sauté the frozen vegetables in the olive oil until tender. Add baked beans and stir well.

3 Pour all of the ingredients into a large deep casserole dish. Bake for about 1 1/2–2 hours at 300°F.

Exchanges
2 Starch
1 Vegetable

Calories 178
Calories from Fat........... 22
Total Fat .... 2 g
Saturated Fat............... 0.4 g
Trans Fat .... 0 g
Cholesterol .... 0 mg
Sodium..........................418 mg
Total Carbohydrate ..... 34 g
Dietary Fiber .... 6 g
Sugars ....17 g
Protein .... 6 g

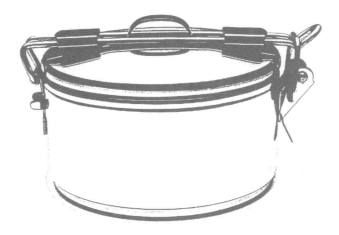

Baked Potatoes

Preparation time: 20 min ✦ Serves 8 ✦ Serving size: 1/3 cup

4	medium potatoes, peeled and cut into 1/4-inch slices
1	cup reduced-fat ranch salad dressing
1/4	tsp salt
1/4	tsp pepper
1/3	cup dry bread crumbs

Toss the potatoes with the ranch dressing, salt, and pepper. Place in a greased 13 × 9 × 2-inch baking pan. Sprinkle with the bread crumbs. Cover and bake at 375°F for 30 minutes. Uncover and bake for 20 more minutes or until potatoes are tender.

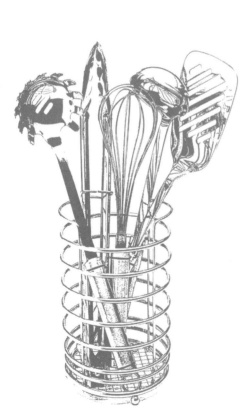

Exchanges
1 1/2 Starch
1/2 Fat

Calories............................144
    Calories from Fat............ 39
Total Fat .... 4 g
    Saturated Fat................. 0.6 g
    Trans Fat .... 0 g
Cholesterol .... 10 mg
Sodium........................... 458 mg
Total Carbohydrate ..... 22 g
    Dietary Fiber .... 2 g
    Sugars .... 3 g
Protein .... 2 g

Broccoli Salad

Preparation time: 30 min ✦ Serves 8 ✦ Serving size: 1/8 recipe

- 2 large heads broccoli
- 1 medium red onion, diced
- 3/4 cup cranberries dried, reserve 1/4 cup
- 1 cup fat-free mayonnaise
- 2 Tbsp nonfat milk
- 2 Tbsp apple cider vinegar
- 1/2 cup Splenda® Sugar Blend for Baking
- 1/3 cup sunflower seeds or chopped walnuts

Clean, trim, and chop the broccoli into a large bowl. Add the diced onion and 1/2 cup dried cranberries. In a separate bowl, mix the mayonnaise, milk, vinegar, Splenda®; stir until smooth. Pour this dressing over the broccoli. Pour into a decorative bowl and garnish with ¼ cup cranberries and sunflower seeds or chopped walnuts. Cover and refrigerate. Serve cold. This recipe is a great source of fiber!

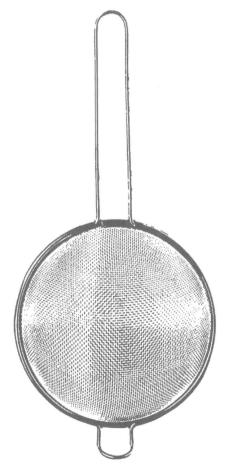

Exchanges
1/2 Fruit
1 Carbohydrate
2 Vegetable
1/2 Fat

Calories..........................191
   Calories from Fat............31
Total Fat ....3 g
   Saturated Fat...............0.3 g
   Trans Fat ....0 g
Cholesterol ....0 mg
Sodium.........................258 mg
Total Carbohydrate ......37 g
   Dietary Fiber ....5 g
   Sugars ....25 g
Protein ....5 g

Cranberry Sauce

Preparation time: 20 min ✦ Serves 50 ✦ Serving size: 2 oz

- 8 cups cranberries
- 2 cups water
- 1 cup Splenda® Sugar Blend for Baking
- 2 cans (11 oz each) mandarin oranges, drained

Combine cranberries and water in a large pot and bring to a boil. Add Splenda® and continue to boil for 2 minutes. Reduce heat and let water and cranberries reduce. After 10 minutes, add the drained mandarin oranges. Remove from heat and cool. Serve with smoked poultry.

Exchanges
1/2 Fruit

Calories	26	
Calories from Fat	0	
Total Fat	0	g
Saturated Fat	0	g
Trans Fat	0	g
Cholesterol	0	mg
Sodium	1	mg
Total Carbohydrate	6	g
Dietary Fiber	1	g
Sugars	6	g
Protein	0	g

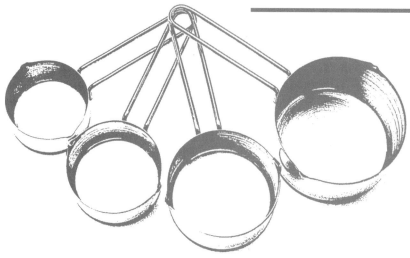

Fried Green Tomatoes

Preparation time: 10 min ✦ Serves 6 ✦ Serving size: 3 tomato slices

1	Tbsp Creole seasoning
1/2	cup egg substitute
1/4	cup low-fat (1%) milk
4	green tomatoes, sliced into 6 pieces per tomato
1/2	cup all-purpose flour
1/2	cup cornmeal
1/4	cup olive oil

Combine the Creole seasoning, egg substitute, and milk in a shallow bowl. Add the tomato slices and let stand for 8 minutes. Combine the flour and cornmeal. Dredge the tomato slices in the flour mixture. Heat the oil in a large skillet and panfry the tomato slices for 4 minutes over medium heat until brown on both sides. Drain on paper towels. Serve warm.

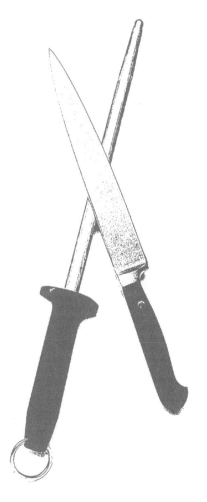

Exchanges
1 Starch
1 Vegetable
2 Fat

Calories	193	
Calories from Fat	86	
Total Fat	10	g
Saturated Fat	1.3	g
Trans Fat	0	g
Cholesterol	1	mg
Sodium	355	mg
Total Carbohydrate	22	g
Dietary Fiber	2	g
Sugars	4	g
Protein	5	g

Fried Rice

Preparation time: 15 min ✦ Serves 8 ✦ Serving size: 3/4 cup

2	Tbsp canola oil
1	medium onion, diced
1/4	tsp salt
1/4	tsp pepper
2-inch piece	fresh ginger, peeled and finely chopped
1 1/3	cups (6 oz) frozen vegetable medley (corn, peas, and carrots)
4	cups cold cooked long-grain rice, white rice, or jasmine rice, grains separated
3	whole scallions, thinly sliced on the bias
3	cloves garlic, finely chopped

1 Heat a nonstick wok over high heat. When hot, add 1 Tbsp of the oil. Add the onion to the wok and season with salt, pepper, and ginger. Cook until the onion is fragrant, about 30 seconds. Add the frozen vegetables. Cook until just defrosted but still crisp. Transfer the contents of the wok to a large bowl.

2 Return the pan to the heat and add the remaining oil. Add the rice to the pan and use a spoon to break up any clumps. Season with salt and pepper, and stir-fry the rice, so it becomes evenly coated with oil. Stop stirring and then let the rice cook until its gets slightly crispy, about 2 minutes. Stir the rice again, breaking up any new clumps. Add the scallions, garlic, and onion vegetable mixture. Stir all the ingredients together with the rice, taste and adjust the seasoning with salt and pepper, if necessary. Serve.

Exchanges
1 1/2 Starch
1 Vegetable
1/2 Fat

Calories	159	
Calories from Fat	33	
Total Fat	4	g
Saturated Fat	0.3	g
Trans Fat	0	g
Cholesterol	0	mg
Sodium	89	mg
Total Carbohydrate	28	g
Dietary Fiber	1	g
Sugars	2	g
Protein	3	g

Glazed Turnips

Preparation time: 30 min ✦ Serves 4 ✦ Serving size: 1/2 cup

2 1/2 cups diced turnips
1 Tbsp olive oil
3 Tbsp Splenda® No Calorie Sweetener
1/4 tsp ground nutmeg
Salt and black pepper to taste

Place the diced turnips in saucepan and boil until almost tender. Drain. Over medium heat, pour the olive oil on the turnips and lightly sauté. Add the Splenda®, nutmeg, and salt and pepper to taste. Cook and stir frequently until turnips are lightly brown and tender.

Exchanges
1 Vegetable
1/2 Fat

Calories........................... 55
　Calories from Fat............31
Total Fat .... 3　g
　Saturated Fat............... 0.5　g
　Trans Fat .... 0　g
Cholesterol .... 0　mg
Sodium........................... 15　mg
Total Carbohydrate .... 6　g
　Dietary Fiber .... 2　g
　Sugars .... 4　g
Protein .... 1　g

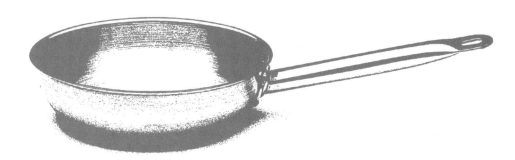

Oliver Greene's Cobb Salad

Preparation time: 15 min ✦ Serves 4 ✦ Serving size: 1 1/2 cups

8	cups baby spinach leaves
1/2	medium red onion, sliced and separated into rings
1	can (11 oz) mandarin oranges, drained
1 1/2	cups sweetened dried cranberries
1/2	cup sliced almonds or pecan halves
1/2	cup fat-free feta cheese, crumbled
1/2	cup balsamic vinaigrette salad dressing

Place servings of spinach onto salad plates. Top with red onion, mandarin oranges, cranberries, sliced almonds, and feta cheese in that order. Drizzle dressing over each salad.

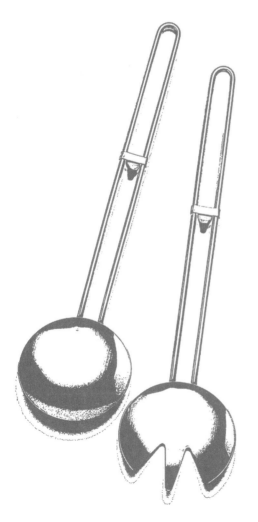

Exchanges
1 1/2 Fruit
1 Vegetable
1 Very Lean Meat
2 1/2 Fat

Calories 268
   Calories from Fat 131
Total Fat .... 15 g
   Saturated Fat .... 1.4 g
   Trans Fat .... 0 g
Cholesterol .... 0 mg
Sodium .... 638 mg
Total Carbohydrate ..... 27 g
   Dietary Fiber .... 5 g
   Sugars .... 19 g
Protein .... 9 g

Grown Folk Spinach Salad

Preparation time: 20 min ✦ Serves 8 ✦ Serving size: 1 medium salad

4	oz turkey bacon, diced
1/4	cup canola oil
1/2	cup finely chopped red onions
1	tsp minced garlic
1/4	tsp freshly ground black pepper
	Pinch salt
1 1/2	Tbsp Creole mustard
1/4	cup red wine vinegar
2	Tbsp sugar
1/2	cup dried cranberries
8	cups fresh spinach, stems removed, washed, and dried (about 12 oz)
1	cup mandarin oranges
2	oz goat cheese, crumbled

1 In a microwave, cook the bacon. Drain on paper towels.

2 Add half of the oil to the skillet and heat. Add the onions and cook, stirring, over medium-high heat until soft, about 3 minutes. Add the garlic, pepper, and salt. Cook, stirring constantly, for 30 seconds. Add the mustard and vinegar and cook, stirring to deglaze the pan. Add the sugar and stir to dissolve. Add the cranberries and cook, stirring, until slightly plumped and warmed through, about 1 minute. Remove from the heat and whisk in the remaining oil. Return the bacon to the pan and adjust the seasoning to taste.

3 In a large bowl, toss the spinach with the warm dressing. Divide the salad among eight salad plates, arrange the orange segments around the edges, crumble the goat cheese over the top, and serve.

Exchanges
1/2 Fruit
1 Vegetable
1 1/2 Fat

Calories	120	
Calories from Fat	55	
Total Fat	6	g
Saturated Fat	1.3	g
Trans Fat	0	g
Cholesterol	0	mg
Sodium	187	mg
Total Carbohydrate	14	g
Dietary Fiber	2	g
Sugars	12	g
Protein	4	g

Mango Salad

Preparation time: 30 min ✦ Serves 12 ✦ Serving size: 1 cup

- 1 cup water
- 1/3 cup Splenda® No Calorie Sweetener
- 1/4 cup lime juice
- 5 small ripe mangoes, peeled and cubed
- 2 cups fresh or water-packed chunk pineapple
- 4 medium bananas, sliced
  Coconut flakes (optional)

Mix the water, Splenda®, and lime juice together in a bowl. Stir until the sugar is completely dissolved. Place the mangoes, pineapple, and bananas in a large bowl. Pour the lime mixture over the fruit. Cover and allow the mixture to chill for 1–2 hours. If desired, garnish with coconut flakes.

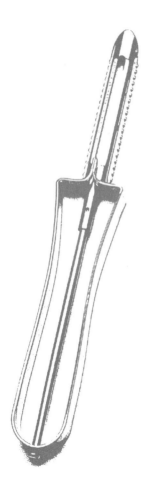

Exchanges
2 Fruit

Calories 128
   Calories from Fat............ 4
Total Fat .... 0 g
   Saturated Fat................... 0 g
   Trans Fat .... 0 g
Cholesterol .... 0 mg
Sodium .... 3 mg
Total Carbohydrate ..... 33 g
   Dietary Fiber .... 3 g
   Sugars .... 26 g
Protein .... 1 g

Mashed Potatoes

Preparation time: 15 min ✦ Serves 16 ✦ Serving size: 1/2 cup

    5   lb potatoes, mashed and cooked
    1   Tbsp garlic, minced
    4   oz fat-free cream cheese
  1/2   cup low-fat (1%) milk
    1   Tbsp light, soft, tub margarine
  1/2   tsp salt

Cook the potatoes until tender. Place hot potatoes in a mixing bowl and add all of the ingredients. Mix well with beaters until smooth. Serve warm.

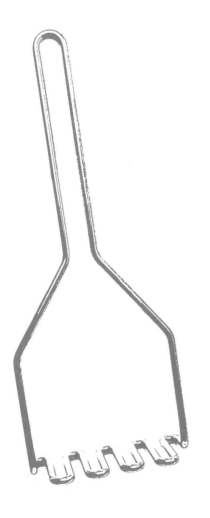

Exchanges
1 1/2 Starch

Calories	111	
Calories from Fat	7	
Total Fat	1	g
Saturated Fat	0.1	g
Trans Fat	0	g
Cholesterol	1	mg
Sodium	143	mg
Total Carbohydrate	23	g
Dietary Fiber	2	g
Sugars	2	g
Protein	3	g

Mix 'N' Mash Potatoes

Preparation time: 1 hour ✦ Serves 8 ✦ Serving size: 1/2 cup

3	medium white potatoes
3	medium sweet potatoes
1/2	cup evaporated nonfat milk
2	Tbsp light, soft, tub margarine
1/8	tsp salt
	White pepper to taste

Scrub the potatoes and place them in a large pot of boiling water. Boil until tender. Drain and cool. Peel all potatoes and mash with a potato masher. Add the milk, margarine, and salt. Cream the potatoes until smooth in texture. Add white pepper to taste.

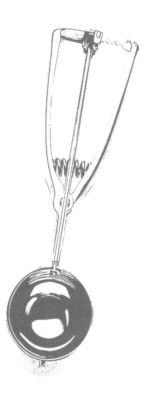

Exchanges
1 1/2 Starch

Calories.........................111
   Calories from Fat.......... 12
Total Fat .... 1 g
   Saturated Fat...............0.1 g
   Trans Fat .... 0 g
Cholesterol .... 0 mg
Sodium........................... 89 mg
Total Carbohydrate ..... 22 g
   Dietary Fiber .... 2 g
   Sugars .... 5 g
Protein .... 3 g

Mixed Greens and Pecan Salad

Preparation time: 10 min ✦ Serves 8 ✦ Serving size: 1/8 recipe

2	lb fresh spinach
1/4	tsp white pepper
4	scallions, thinly sliced, including about 2 inches of the green part
3	Tbsp olive oil
1/4	cup lemon juice
1/4	cup pecans, toasted and chopped

Put the spinach in a salad bowl and sprinkle it with pepper. Add the scallions to the bowl. Pour on the olive oil and toss the salad thoroughly. Add the lemon juice and toss. Top with the pecans and serve. You can also blend the dressing ingredients in the blender, creating a temporary emulsion.

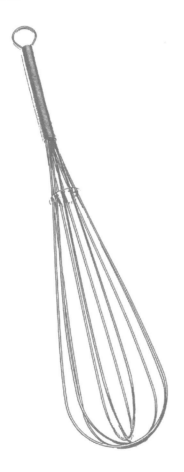

Exchanges
1 Vegetable
2 Fat

Calories 126
    Calories from Fat 98
Total Fat .... 11 g
    Saturated Fat .... 1.2 g
    Trans Fat .... 0 g
Cholesterol .... 0 mg
Sodium .... 93 mg
Total Carbohydrate .... 6 g
    Dietary Fiber .... 3 g
    Sugars .... 1 g
Protein .... 4 g

Peas and Rice

Preparation time: 10 min ✦ Serves 16 ✦ Serving size: 1/2 cup

2	Tbsp olive oil
1	large onion, chopped
2	cups white rice, uncooked
2	tsp turmeric
1	quart reduced-sodium, low-fat chicken broth
1 1/2	cup frozen peas and carrots
	Salt and pepper to taste (*optional*)

In a large Dutch oven, heat the oil and chopped onions and sauté until soft. Add the rice and turmeric; stir to coat rice. Add the chicken broth, bring to a quick boil, and then reduce to a simmer. Cook until the rice absorbs all of the broth. Stir to prevent sticking. Stir in thawed vegetables. Simmer for 10 minutes. Add salt and pepper to taste.

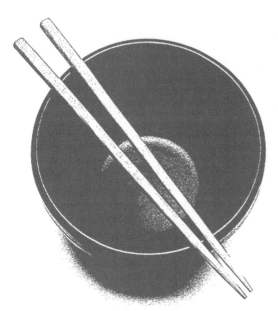

Exchanges
1 1/2 Starch

Calories 127
    Calories from Fat............18
Total Fat .... 2 g
    Saturated Fat................ 0.3 g
    Trans Fat .... 0 g
Cholesterol .... 0 mg
Sodium ....137 mg
Total Carbohydrate ..... 23 g
    Dietary Fiber .... 1 g
    Sugars .... 2 g
Protein .... 3 g

Power Salad

Preparation time: 30 min ✦ Serves 8 ✦ Serving size: 1/2 cup

4	medium sweet potatoes
4	medium green apples
2	Tbsp lime juice
2	Tbsp Splenda® No Calorie Sweetener
3	Tbsp raisins
4	Tbsp chopped walnuts
1/4	tsp salt
1/2	cup nonfat yogurt
3	Tbsp reduced-fat mayonnaise

1 Wash and peel the sweet potatoes. Cut into 1-inch cubes and place in a vegetable steamer. Steam over boiling water for 15 minutes until tender, but firm. Cool the sweet potatoes. Wash the apples, remove seeds, and cut into 1-inch cubes. Sprinkle with lime juice and Splenda®. In a large bowl, combine the raisins, walnuts, salt, sweet potatoes, and apples.

2 In a separate bowl, combine the yogurt with the mayonnaise. Mix well and toss into the sweet potato mix.

Exchanges
1 Starch
1 Fruit
1 Fat

Calories..........................166	
Calories from Fat...........41	
Total Fat 5	g
Saturated Fat................0.6	g
Trans Fat 0	g
Cholesterol 2	mg
Sodium..........................140	mg
Total Carbohydrate 31	g
Dietary Fiber 3	g
Sugars 15	g
Protein 3	g

Rainbow Salsa

Preparation time: 15 min ✦ Serves 8 ✦ Serving size: 1/4 cup

1	15-oz can canned black beans, rinsed and drained
1 1/2	cup yellow corn, fresh or frozen
1	cup chopped red bell pepper, minced
1	cup green bell pepper, chopped
1/2	medium purple onion, finely chopped
1	Tbsp fresh parsley
1/2	cup reduced-fat sour cream
1/4	cup fat-free mayonnaise
3	Tbsp red wine vinegar
1	tsp cumin
1	tsp chili powder
1/2	tsp salt
1/4	tsp garlic powder
1/8	tsp pepper

In a large bowl, combine the beans, corn, bell peppers, onions, and parsley. In a separate bowl, combine the sour cream and mayonnaise and mix well. Add vinegar and seasonings. Pour over bean mixture. Coat well.

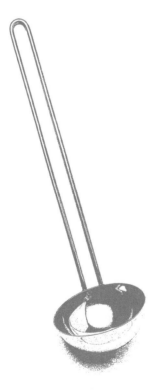

Exchanges
1 Starch
1 Vegetable

Calories........................110
   Calories from Fat............16
Total Fat .... 2 g
   Saturated Fat................1.1 g
   Trans Fat .... 0 g
Cholesterol .... 6 mg
Sodium......................... 263 mg
Total Carbohydrate ..... 20 g
   Dietary Fiber .... 4 g
   Sugars .... 5 g
Protein .... 5 g

Raspberry-Cranberry Relish

Preparation time: 20 min ✦ Serves 8 ✦ Serving size: 1/8 recipe

1 1/2	lb cranberries, fresh or frozen
2	pints raspberries
	Pinch ground cinnamon
1/2	cup water
1	medium orange, well washed
1/2	cup orange marmalade
1/2	cup unsweetened applesauce
2	Tbsp fresh lemon juice

1 In a heavy, nonreactive saucepan, combine the cranberries, raspberries, and cinnamon in the water. Carefully remove the peel from the orange, leaving behind the white pith. Finely slice the peel into thin strips and add it to the cranberries. Remove the pith from the orange, reserving the orange.

2 Bring the cranberries to a boil over medium heat. Reduce the heat and simmer. Add the orange marmalade, stirring until the cranberries are cooked and the sugar has dissolved, about 8–10 minutes. Remove from heat and let cool slightly. Segment the reserved orange, discard the membranes and any seeds, and place it in a food processor. Chop until pulpy. Stir the orange into the cranberries; add the applesauce and lemon juice.

3 Transfer the sauce to a container and refrigerate overnight before serving.

Exchanges
2 1/2 Fruit

Calories.........................139	
Calories from Fat............ 5	
Total Fat 1	g
Saturated Fat.................. 0	g
Trans Fat 0	g
Cholesterol 0	mg
Sodium...........................14	mg
Total Carbohydrate 36	g
Dietary Fiber 9	g
Sugars 25	g
Protein 1	g

Red Tofu with Mushrooms

Preparation time: 20 min ✦ Serves 6 ✦ Serving size: 6 oz

2	12-oz (24 oz total) blocks of firm or extra-firm tofu, cut into 1-inch squares
1	Tbsp paprika
1	tsp cayenne pepper (*optional*)
1 1/2	tsp kosher salt
1	Tbsp safflower oil, peanut oil, or grapeseed oil
3	bunches scallions, chopped
12	cloves garlic, crushed
1	pint Shitake mushrooms or white button mushrooms
30	broccoli florets, cut into bite-size pieces
2	Tbsp rice vinegar
1	Tbsp water
30	whole basil leaves

Mushroom sauce

1/4	cup water
6	shiitake or white button mushrooms
2	tsp rice vinegar
1/2	tsp arrowroot

1 Before cutting the tofu into squares, season it by sprinkling a light coat of paprika, cayenne, and a pinch of salt on one side of each block of tofu. Place the block on its side and cut into 1-inch slices.

2 In a hot skillet (cast iron), heat the oil. Lay the sheets of tofu, seasoned side down first. Add the scallions, crushed garlic cloves, mushrooms, and broccoli florets. Once you finish adding all of the vegetables, flip the tofu and give the pan a good shake or use a wooden spoon to stir the vegetables.

3 Add the rice vinegar and water (or substitute a white wine, such as pinot grigio or sauvignon blanc) and cover. Turn the heat down to medium to finish steaming the broccoli, about 1–2 minutes. Garnish each dish with basil leaves.

4 In a blender, prepare the mushroom sauce. Combine the water, mushrooms, and rice vinegar and puree until smooth. Add arrowroot to puree and blend until thickened. This dish can be served alone or with a meat.

Exchanges
2 Vegetable
1 Medium-Fat Meat
1/2 Fat

Calories 153
  Calories from Fat 69
Total Fat .... 8 g
  Saturated Fat .... 1.1 g
  Trans Fat .... 0 g
Cholesterol .... 0 mg
Sodium .... 519 mg
Total Carbohydrate ..... 13 g
  Dietary Fiber .... 5 g
  Sugars .... 4 g
Protein .... 13 g

Roasted Rutabaga with Caramelized Onions

Preparation time: 30 min ✦ Serves 6 ✦ Serving size: 1/4 cup

Rutabaga
1/2 Tbsp olive oil
1 medium rutabaga (about 1 lb)
1/2 tsp salt

Caramelized onions
1 tsp canola oil
2 medium onions, thinly sliced lengthwise
1/4 tsp salt
Fresh ground pepper to taste
Garnish: coarsely chopped cilantro

1 Rub the olive oil over outer core of rutabaga, making sure to cover all of it. Sprinkle with salt and wrap in aluminum foil. Bake in an oven at 350°F for 1 hour or until tender.

2 Meanwhile, in a large saucepan, combine the oil, onions, salt, and pepper. Cover and cook over medium-low heat, until the onions are clear and soft, about 5 minutes. Uncover and increase heat to medium and sauté. Stir and toss frequently, until the onions are brown. Garnish with cilantro.

3 Remove the rutabaga from the oven and peel away the wax covering with large knife. Cut it into small wedges and arrange on platter. Spread caramelized onions on top.

Exchanges
2 Vegetable
1/2 Fat

Calories...........................61		
Calories from Fat............18		
Total Fat 2	g	
Saturated Fat............... 0.2	g	
Trans Fat 0	g	
Cholesterol 0	mg	
Sodium......................... 304	mg	
Total Carbohydrate 10	g	
Dietary Fiber 2	g	
Sugars 6	g	
Protein 1	g	

Spicy Plantains

Preparation time: 15 min ✦ Serves 6 ✦ Serving size: 1/6 recipe

- 4 large ripe plantains
- 2 Tbsp water, add more as needed
- 1 tsp fresh ground ginger
- 1/2 tsp salt
- 1/2 tsp cayenne pepper

Peel and slice the plantains into 1-inch-thick pieces. Soak plantains in a small bowl with water, ginger, salt, and cayenne pepper. Make sure the plantains are evenly coated. Drain liquid and steam plantains until tender.

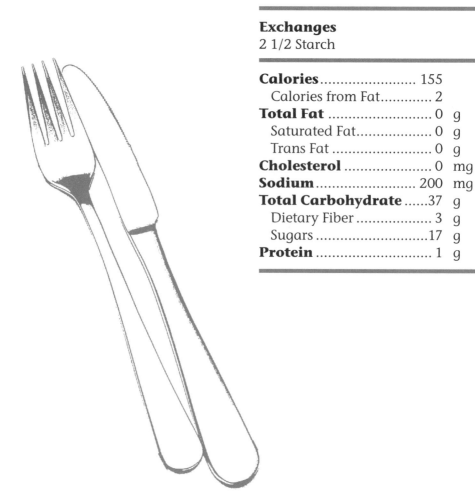

Exchanges
2 1/2 Starch

Calories 155
   Calories from Fat 2
Total Fat .... 0 g
   Saturated Fat .... 0 g
   Trans Fat .... 0 g
Cholesterol .... 0 mg
Sodium .... 200 mg
Total Carbohydrate ...... 37 g
   Dietary Fiber .... 3 g
   Sugars .... 17 g
Protein .... 1 g

Spicy Zucchini Quesadillas

Preparation time: 20 min ✦ Serves 8 ✦ Serving size: 1 quesadilla

1	large onion, chopped
1/2	cup chopped sweet red pepper
2	tsp olive oil
2	cups julienned zucchini
2	Tbsp taco seasoning
8	flour tortillas (7 inches each)
1/4	cup fat-free cheddar cheese, shredded
3	Tbsp salsa
1/2	cup fat-free sour cream
1/2	cup pickled jalapeno pepper slices

1 In a skillet, sauté the onion and red pepper in olive oil for 3 minutes. Stir in the zucchini and taco seasoning; sauté for 3–4 minutes longer or until vegetables are tender. Remove from heat.

2 Heat the tortillas in a nonstick pan or in the oven at 300°F. Sprinkle a pinch of cheese and 1/4 cup of zucchini mixture over half of each tortilla and then fold over.

3 Cook over low heat for 1–2 minutes on each side or until cheese is melted. Serve with salsa, sour cream, and jalapenos.

Exchanges
1 1/2 Starch
2 Vegetable
1 Fat

Calories	204	
Calories from Fat	44	
Total Fat	5	g
Saturated Fat	1.1	g
Trans Fat	0	g
Cholesterol	2	mg
Sodium	708	mg
Total Carbohydrate	31	g
Dietary Fiber	3	g
Sugars	4	g
Protein	8	g

Squash Casserole

Preparation time: 20 min ✦ Serves 8 ✦ Serving size: 1/2 cup

  1 1/2 lb summer squash
     2 Tbsp light, soft, tub margarine, melted
   1/2 pkg (about 7 oz) herbed cubed stuffing mix
     1 10.75-oz can 98% fat-free, reduced-sodium cream of chicken soup
     1 4-oz jar pimientos, drained
     1 medium onion, chopped
     1 cup carrots, grated
     1 cup fat-free sour cream

1 Cook the squash in boiling water. Drain and mash. In a separate bowl, mix the margarine with the stuffing mix. Set aside. Combine the remaining ingredients with the mashed squash.

2 Use half of the stuffing mixture to line the bottom of the casserole dish; spread squash mixture over the stuffing mix.

3 Use the other half of the stuffing mix to cover the top of squash mixture. Bake at 350°F for 35 minutes.

Exchanges
1 1/2 Starch
2 Vegetable
1/2 Fat

Calories 191
   Calories from Fat 30
Total Fat .... 3 g
   Saturated Fat .... 0.5 g
   Trans Fat .... 0 g
Cholesterol .... 7 mg
Sodium .... 618 mg
Total Carbohydrate ..... 32 g
   Dietary Fiber .... 4 g
   Sugars .... 7 g
Protein .... 7 g

Strawberry Soup

Preparation time: 25 min ✦ Serves 8 ✦ Serving size: 1/2 cup

4	cups fresh strawberries
1/2	cup apple juice
3/4	cup water
1/4	cup Splenda® Sugar Blend for Baking
	Pinch ground cloves
3	6-oz containers nonfat yogurt
	Red food coloring (optional)
	Strawberry halves (optional)

1 In a saucepan, combine 2 cups strawberries, apple juice, water, Splenda®, and cloves; bring to a boil over medium heat. Remove from heat and allow to cool. Strain the strawberry broth, discarding the cooked berries only.

2 Place 2 cups fresh (uncooked) strawberries and 1/3 cup of the strawberry broth in a blender or food processor; cover and process until smooth. Pour into large bowl. Add the remaining broth, yogurt, and red food coloring, if desired. Cover. Refrigerate until well chilled. Garnish with additional strawberries, if desired.

Exchanges
1 Carbohydrate

Calories	69	
Calories from Fat	2	
Total Fat	0	g
Saturated Fat	0	g
Trans Fat	0	g
Cholesterol	1	mg
Sodium	32	mg
Total Carbohydrate	15	g
Dietary Fiber	1	g
Sugars	13	g
Protein	2	g

Sweet Potato Mash

Preparation time: 20 min ✦ Serves 18 ✦ Serving size: 1/3 cup

5	lb sweet potatoes
3/4	cup evaporated nonfat milk
3	Tbsp light, soft, tub margarine
1/2	tsp salt
1/2	tsp cinnamon
1/4	tsp nutmeg
	Nonstick cooking spray
1/2	cup Splenda® Brown Sugar Blend
1/4	cup chopped pecans

1 Boil or bake the sweet potatoes until soft. While sweet potatoes are still hot, peel them and mash.

2 Combine all ingredients in a large bowl, except the Splenda® and pecans. Pour the mixture into an 11 × 7-inch baking dish sprayed with nonstick cooking spray. Sprinkle the Splenda® and pecans on top. Broil for a few minutes until sugar melts. Remove from heat and let stand.

Exchanges
2 Starch

Calories	168	
Calories from Fat	20	
Total Fat	2	g
Saturated Fat	0.2	g
Trans Fat	0	g
Cholesterol	0	mg
Sodium	108	mg
Total Carbohydrate	33	g
Dietary Fiber	2	g
Sugars	13	g
Protein	3	g

Taters

Preparation time: 25 min ✦ Serves 8 ✦ Serving size: 1/8 recipe

6	medium sweet potatoes, cooked and peeled
1/4	cup flour
2	Tbsp canola oil
1/4	cup Splenda® Brown Sugar Blend
1/2	tsp salt
1/2	tsp nutmeg

1 Cut the cooked sweet potatoes into 1/2-inch strips. Coat each with flour. Heat oil to 365°F in a skillet on medium heat. Panfry the potato fingers for 4–5 minutes or until golden brown.

2 Combine Splenda®, salt, and nutmeg. Sprinkle over sweet potatoes. Toss lightly until sugar melts. Serve hot.

Exchanges
2 Starch
1/2 Fat

Calories	173	
Calories from Fat	34	
Total Fat	4	g
Saturated Fat	0.3	g
Trans Fat	0	g
Cholesterol	0	mg
Sodium	161	mg
Total Carbohydrate	33	g
Dietary Fiber	2	g
Sugars	12	g
Protein	2	g

Tomato and Onion Salad

Preparation time: 5 min ✦ Serves 4 ✦ Serving size: 1 tomato

        4 large tomatoes
        1 large Vidalia onion, thinly sliced
     1/2 cup fat-free red wine vinaigrette dressing
        2 oz reduced-fat mozzarella cheese, cut into strips or cubes
            Garnish: fresh basil, chopped

Slice tomatoes into wedges. Combine remaining ingredients in a separate bowl. Place tomatoes on separate plates, spoon onion mixture on top. Serve chilled. Garnish with fresh chopped basil.

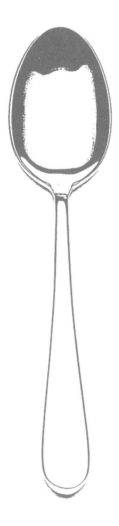

Exchanges
3 Vegetable
1/2 Fat

Calories	96
Calories from Fat	22
Total Fat	2 g
Saturated Fat	1.3 g
Trans Fat	0 g
Cholesterol	8 mg
Sodium	111 mg
Total Carbohydrate	15 g
Dietary Fiber	3 g
Sugars	9 g
Protein	6 g

Trash-Talkin' Grilled Tofu Steaks

Preparation time: 20 min ✦ Serves 6 ✦ Serving size: 4 oz

24	oz firm tofu
1	Tbsp paprika
2	tsp cumin
2	tsp garlic powder
2 1/2	tsp chipotle chili pepper
1 1/2	tsp salt
1	medium onion, sliced into rings
2	tsp olive oil spray

1 Place the tofu block on its side and cut into 1 1/2- to 2-inch slices.

2 Combine the paprika, cumin, garlic powder, chipotle chili pepper, and salt in a ramekin to make a rub. Sprinkle a medium to moderate amount of rub on each slice of tofu, making sure to coat both sides. Lightly spray each side of the tofu slices with the olive oil before placing on the grill; doing this will make grill marks on each side.

3 Grill the tofu for 2 1/2 minutes on each side over medium-high heat. Grill the onion slices to serve with the tofu. This dish works best when served with grilled corn on the cob, portabella mushrooms, and asparagus on a bed of green salad.

Exchanges
1 Vegetable
1 Medium-Fat Meat

Calories........................109
   Calories from Fat.......... 54
Total Fat .... 6 g
   Saturated Fat................1.1 g
   Trans Fat .... 0 g
Cholesterol .... 0 mg
Sodium........................ 609 mg
Total Carbohydrate .... 7 g
   Dietary Fiber .... 2 g
   Sugars .... 3 g
Protein .... 10 g

Tri-Color Slaw

Preparation time: 15 min ✦ Serves 12 ✦ Serving size: 1/12 recipe

6	cups ready-cut tri-color cabbage
1	medium red apple
1	medium green apple
1	cup golden raisins
1/4	cup pecans, chopped
1/4	cup honey
1	Tbsp lemon juice
3/4	cup reduced-fat sour cream
1/4	tsp salt
1/8	tsp pepper
1/4	tsp nutmeg

In large bowl, combine the cabbage, apples, raisins, and pecans. In a separate bowl, combine the honey and lemon juice; stir well. Add the sour cream, salt, pepper, and nutmeg. Pour this mix over the cabbage mixture; stir well. Serve cold.

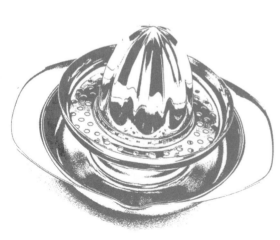

Exchanges
1 Fruit
1/2 Carbohydrate
1/2 Fat

Calories........................117
   Calories from Fat........... 28
Total Fat .... 3 g
   Saturated Fat................ 1.2 g
   Trans Fat .... 0 g
Cholesterol .... 6 mg
Sodium.......................... 69 mg
Total Carbohydrate ..... 22 g
   Dietary Fiber .... 2 g
   Sugars .... 19 g
Protein .... 2 g

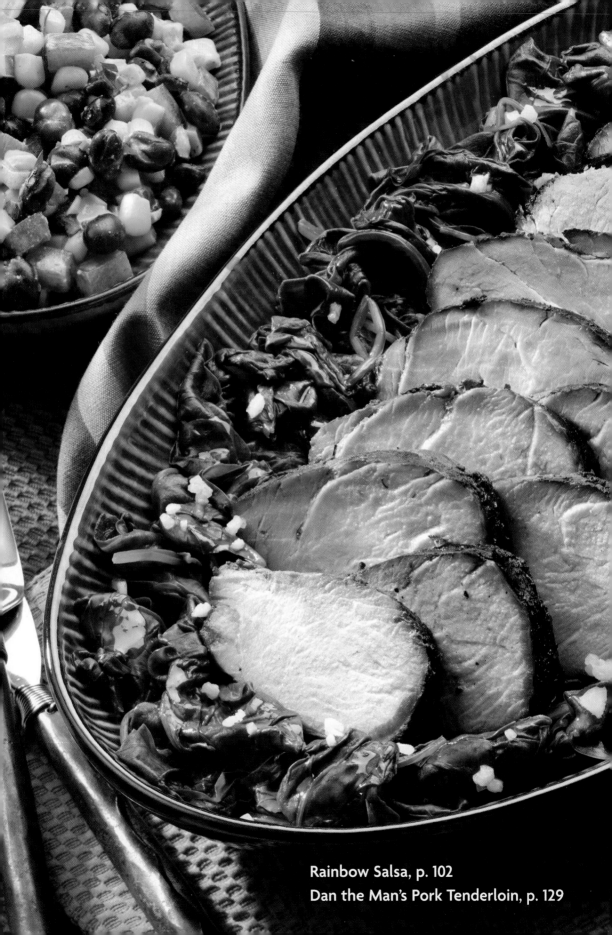

Rainbow Salsa, p. 102
Dan the Man's Pork Tenderloin, p. 129

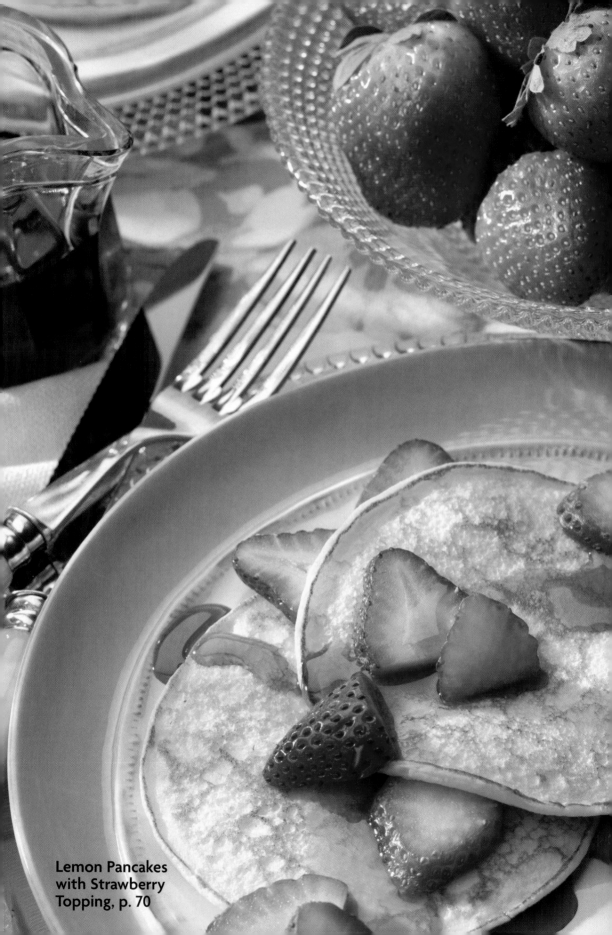

Lemon Pancakes
with Strawberry
Topping, p. 70

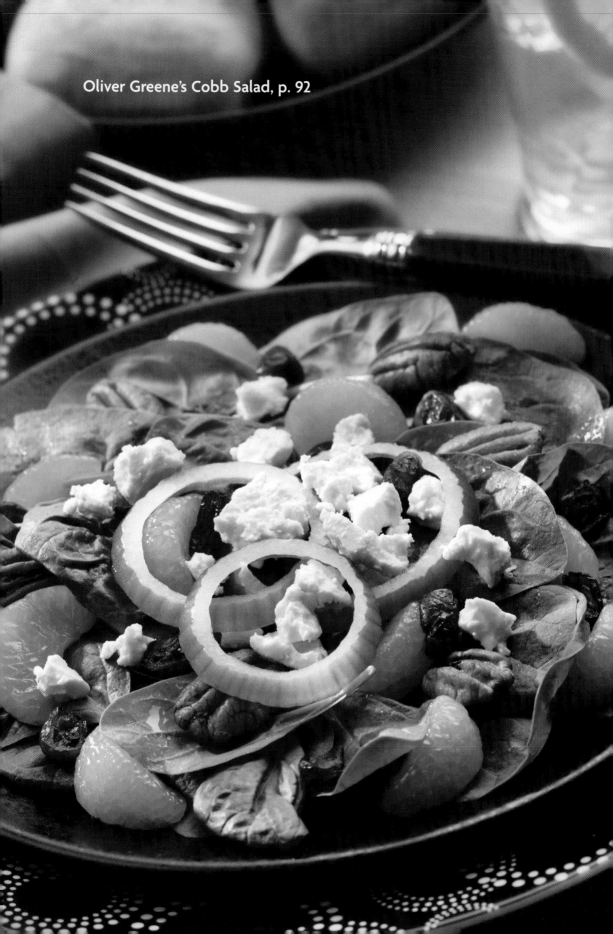
Oliver Greene's Cobb Salad, p. 92

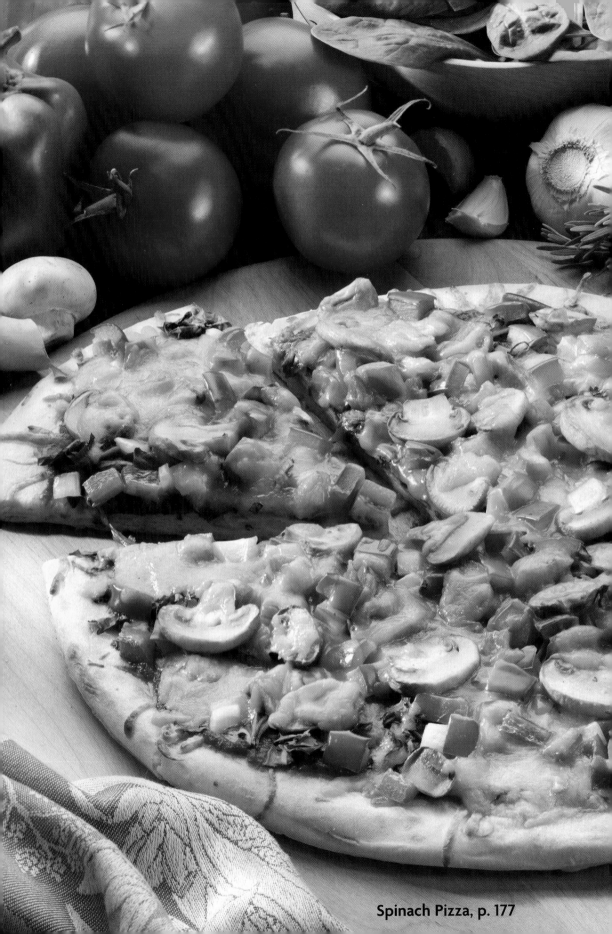

Spinach Pizza, p. 177

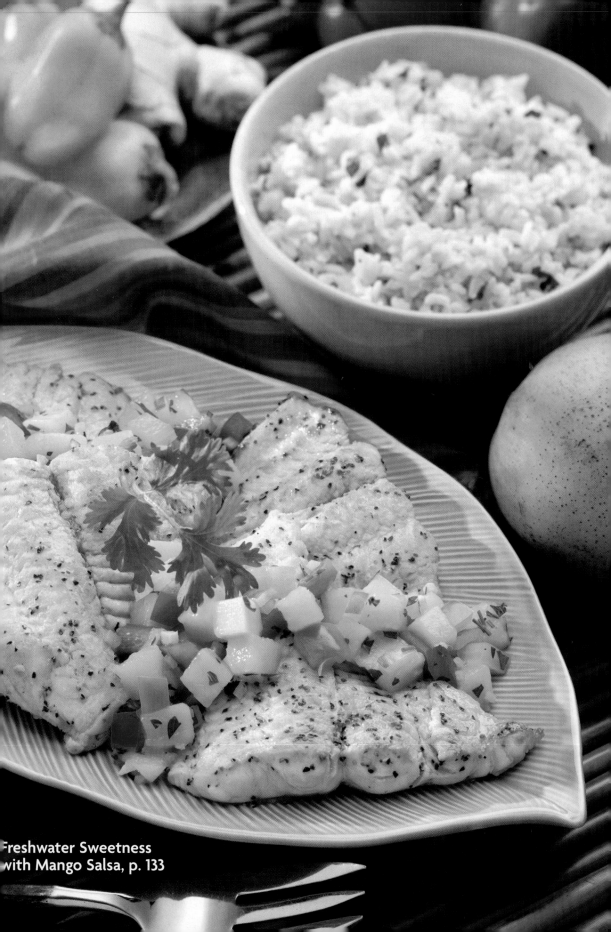

Freshwater Sweetness
with Mango Salsa, p. 133

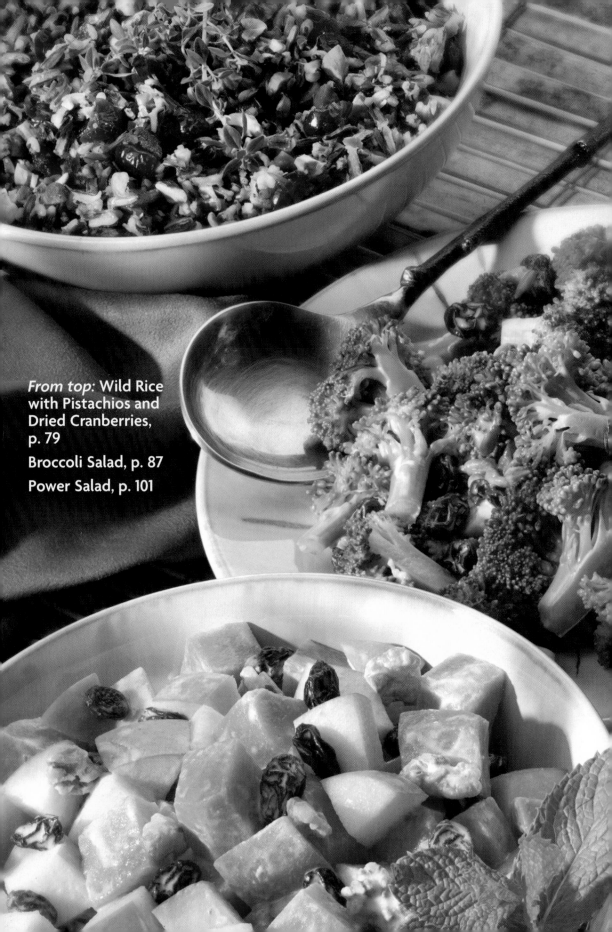

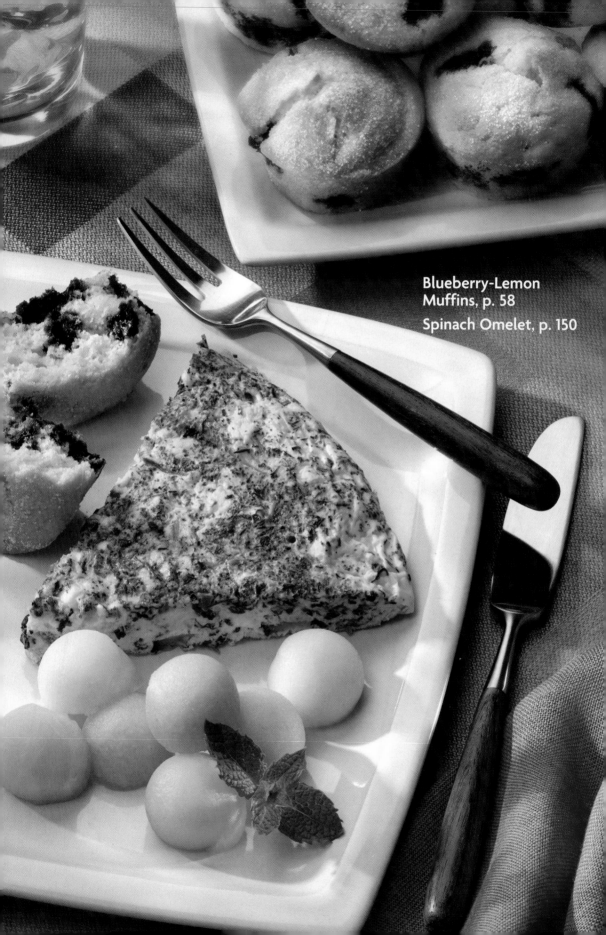

Blueberry-Lemon
Muffins, p. 58

Spinach Omelet, p. 150

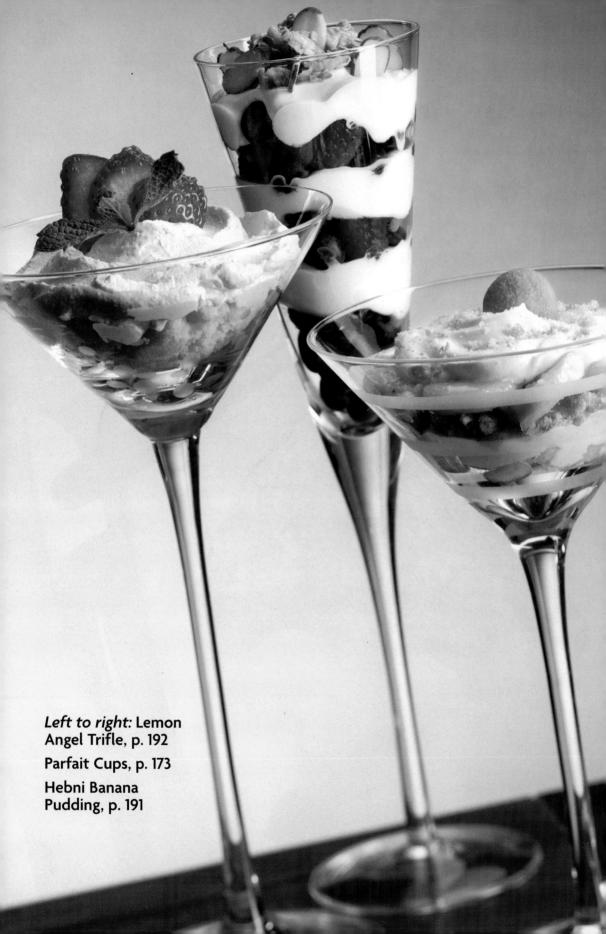

Left to right: **Lemon Angel Trifle, p. 192**

Parfait Cups, p. 173

Hebni Banana Pudding, p. 191

Where's the Beef, Baby!

Preparation time: 25 min ✦ Serves 8 ✦ Serving size: 1 cup

3/4	cup cashew nuts
1	large (7 oz) onion
1	cup green and red bell pepper
1	cup eggplant
2	12-oz blocks (24 oz total) extra-firm tofu, diced
1	Jalapeno pepper, diced
2	Tbsp fresh ginger, grated or chopped fine
1	cup fresh corn
8	large portabella mushrooms
1 1/2	tsp salt
1	Tbsp chipotle chili pepper spice

Garnish: 1 bunch cilantro, rough chopped
1 bunch parsley, rough chopped

1 Toast the raw cashew nuts for 5 minutes at 350°F, and then let cool while preparing the stuffed mushrooms. Once cool, place them in a food processor and pulse the cashews to give them a light chop (or you can use a knife to chop them).

2 Small dice the onion, bell pepper, eggplant, and tofu. Finely chop the jalapeno pepper and the ginger. In a large mixing bowl, place the diced eggplant, green and red bell pepper, corn, onion, and the tofu. Mix thoroughly.

3 Place 1/2 cup of the mixture in each portabella cap, and then sprinkle each cap with a pinch of ginger, jalapeno pepper, salt, and chipotle chili pepper spice. Place on a nonstick sheet and bake for 15–20 minutes at 375°F. Serve hot, garnish with cilantro and parsley.

Roasted Corn Sauce

If you'd like to have a sauce with this dish, you can use or make cream corn and simply spoon a little bit on top of each mushroom cap. Roast 3 whole corncobs for 15 minutes at 350°F. Shave the kernels from the ears and place them in a blender with 1/2 cup water and 1/2 cup white wine. Puree until you get a delicious sauce. (Not included in nutritional analysis.)

Exchanges
1 Starch
3 Vegetable
1 Medium-Fat Meat
1 Fat

Calories......................... 269	
Calories from Fat......... 120	
Total Fat 13	g
Saturated Fat............... 2.3	g
Trans Fat 0	g
Cholesterol 0	mg
Sodium......................... 493	mg
Total Carbohydrate 28	g
Dietary Fiber 5	g
Sugars 8	g
Protein 15	g

Willa's Apple Salad

Preparation time: 10 min ✦ Serves 8 ✦ Serving size: 1/8 recipe

3	medium Granny Smith apples, chopped
2	Tbsp lemon juice
1/2	cup pecans
1/2	cup dried cranberries
1	cup fat-free mayonnaise
1/3	cup red wine vinegar
1	tsp Splenda® No Calorie Sweetener
1	large (9 oz) bag fresh spinach, divided onto four salad plates

Chop the apples and place them in a mixing bowl. Drizzle lemon juice over them to prevent browning. Add the pecans and dried cranberries; mix thoroughly and chill in the refrigerator. In another bowl, combine the mayonnaise, vinegar, and Splenda®. Mix thoroughly to create a smooth dressing. Add dressing to chilled apple mixture; serve on a bed of spinach.

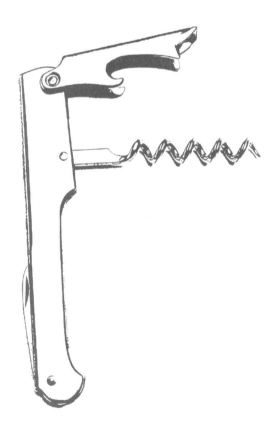

Exchanges
1 1/2 Fruit
1 Fat

Calories 129
 Calories from Fat 49
Total Fat .... 5 g
 Saturated Fat .... 0.5 g
 Trans Fat .... 0 g
Cholesterol .... 0 mg
Sodium .... 237 mg
Total Carbohydrate ..... 20 g
 Dietary Fiber .... 3 g
 Sugars .... 14 g
Protein .... 2 g

Side Dish Salsa

Preparation time: 5 min ✦ Serves 21 ✦ Serving size: 1/4 cup

1	whole cucumber, seeded and chopped
1	cup green bell pepper, diced
1	cup red bell pepper, diced
1/3	cup purple onion, diced
2/3	cup mango or other firm fruit, such as papaya
1/4	tsp salt
	Dash champagne vinegar to taste
1/4	cup cilantro
1–2	Tbsp lime juice
1	tsp Splenda®

Combine all ingredients. Stir well. Adjust cilantro to taste. If you prefer this salsa to taste sweeter, add 1 tsp Splenda®. Refrigerate and serve cold with pork, beef, or fish.

Exchanges
Free Food

Calories 10
   Calories from Fat 1
Total Fat .... 0 g
   Saturated Fat .... 0 g
   Trans Fat .... 0 g
Cholesterol .... 0 mg
Sodium .... 29 mg
Total Carbohydrate .... 2 g
   Dietary Fiber .... 0 g
   Sugars .... 2 g
Protein .... 0 g

Soul Food
Meats

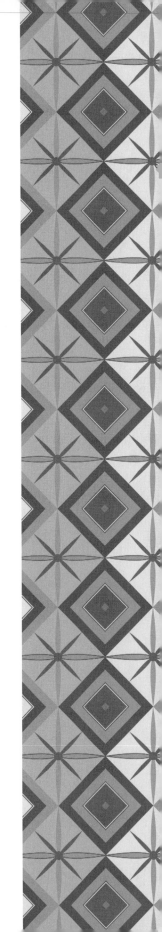

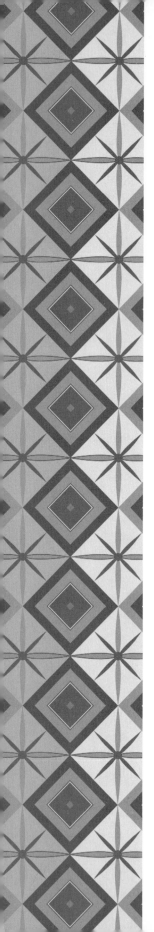

Albacore Stir-Fry

Preparation time: 15 min ✦ Serves 4 ✦ Serving size: 1/4 recipe

- 1   Tbsp canola oil
- 1   cup onion, chopped
- 2   large cloves garlic, minced
- 1   24-oz bag frozen Oriental vegetables
- 2   6-oz cans solid white albacore tuna, packed in water and drained
- 1   Tbsp lite soy sauce
- 1   Tbsp lemon juice
- 1   tsp Splenda® No Calorie Sweetener
- 2   cups cooked brown rice

Heat the oil in a large skillet. Stir in onion, garlic, and frozen vegetables; cook until crisp, about 3 minutes. Add tuna, soy sauce, lemon juice, and Splenda®, and cook for 1 minute. Serve over cooked rice.

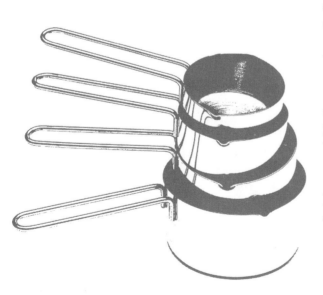

Exchanges
1 1/2 Starch
3 Vegetable
2 Lean Meat

Calories........................ 309
   Calories from Fat........... 44
Total Fat .... 5 g
   Saturated Fat............... 0.6 g
   Trans Fat .... 0 g
Cholesterol .... 23 mg
Sodium........................457 mg
Total Carbohydrate ..... 38 g
   Dietary Fiber .... 6 g
   Sugars .... 9 g
Protein .... 25 g

Baked Fish Fillets with Peppers

Preparation time: 20 min ✦ Serves 6 ✦ Serving size: 1/2 cup

   6 fish fillets, such as catfish, halibut, or walleye, about 1 1/2 lb each
       Nonstick cooking spray
   1 Tbsp olive oil
   1 green bell pepper, cut into strips
   1 red bell pepper, cut into strips
 1/4 tsp chopped ginger
 1/4 tsp curry powder
   1 Tbsp lemon juice

Preheat oven to 400°F. Place the fish fillets on a broiler pan rack coated with nonstick cooking spray; bake for 5 minutes. In a pan, heat the oil. Sauté the peppers and ginger until soft, and then add the curry powder and lemon juice; cook for 2 minutes. Remove the fish fillets from the oven and add to pan. Be sure to coat each fillet with sauce. Cook for 5 minutes or until fish flakes and serve hot.

Exchanges
3 Lean Meat
1/2 Fat

Calories 187
   Calories from Fat 95
Total Fat .... 11 g
   Saturated Fat .... 2.2 g
   Trans Fat .... 0 g
Cholesterol .... 65 mg
Sodium .... 180 mg
Total Carbohydrate .... 3 g
   Dietary Fiber .... 1 g
   Sugars .... 2 g
Protein .... 20 g

Cajun Pirate Shrimp

Preparation time: 20 min ✦ Serves 6 ✦ Serving size: 1/6 recipe

1/2	cup water
1	6-oz can tomato paste
2	Tbsp hot pepper sauce
2	Tbsp Worcestershire sauce
1	Tbsp vegetable oil
1	cup onion, chopped
1	cup celery, chopped
1	16-oz pkg frozen stir-fry vegetables
2	Tbsp water
1/2	lb cooked shrimp
2	cups cooked brown rice
	Garnish: chopped fresh cilantro

1 In a small bowl, combine the water, tomato paste, hot pepper sauce, and Worcestershire sauce. Stir well. Set aside.

2 In a large skillet, heat the oil. Stir-fry the onions and celery until crisp tender. Add frozen vegetables and 2 Tbsp water. Cover and cook for 7–10 minutes.

3 Uncover and stir in reserved sauce mixture. Add cooked shrimp and heat through.

4 Serve over hot rice. Garnish with cilantro, if desired.

Exchanges
1 Starch
3 Vegetable
1 Lean Meat

Calories........................199
　Calories from Fat........... 33
Total Fat .... 4　g
　Saturated Fat................ 0.4　g
　Trans Fat .... 0　g
Cholesterol ....74　mg
Sodium..........................213　mg
Total Carbohydrate ..... 29　g
　Dietary Fiber .... 5　g
　Sugars .... 6　g
Protein .... 12　g

Cat Island Grouper Steaks

Preparation time: 20 min ✦ Serves 4 ✦ Serving size: 1 fillet

 4 grouper fillets (about 5 oz each)
 4 cloves garlic, minced
 1 Scotch bonnet pepper or other hot pepper, seeded and finely chopped (*if this will be too hot for you, just use half of the pepper, but be sure to use rubber or latex gloves to handle the pepper*)
 1/2 tsp salt
 1 tsp freshly ground black pepper
 3/4 cup fresh lime juice
 1 bunch chives or 4 scallions, finely chopped
 2 shallots, thinly sliced
 1 small onion, thinly sliced
 3 Tbsp finely chopped cilantro
 4 sprigs fresh thyme or 1 tsp dried thyme leaves
 4 bay leaves
 1 tsp allspice

1 Rinse the grouper fillets and blot dry. (If you can't find grouper, substitute with red snapper or any other saltwater fish.) Make 3 or 4 small deep slits in the fillet, depending on the thickness of each steak. Arrange the fish in a baking dish just large enough to hold them.

2 Prepare the marinade. Place the garlic, hot pepper, salt, and pepper in the bottom of a mixing bowl and mash to a paste with the back of a spoon. Add the lime juice and stir until the salt crystals are dissolved. Stir in the chives or scallions, shallots, onion, and cilantro. Set aside.

3 In a separate bowl, combine the thyme, bay leaves, and allspice. Spread this mixture on the fish and into the slits of the fillets. Pour the marinade over the fish and marinate in the refrigerator for 1 hour, turning once or twice.

4 Preheat a grill to high heat. Brush the grill with oil. If you are using a fish basket, oil it before placing the fish in it. Arrange on the grill and cook until the fish is done, 6–12 minutes per side (depending on the size of the fish), turning gently with a spatula. Transfer the fish to a clean platter and serve at once.

Exchanges
1/2 Carbohydrate
5 Very Lean Meat

Calories..........................197
 Calories from Fat............18
Total Fat ....2 g
 Saturated Fat...............0.5 g
 Trans Fat ....0 g
Cholesterol ....67 mg
Sodium..........................305 mg
Total Carbohydrate ....7 g
 Dietary Fiber ....1 g
 Sugars ....2 g
Protein ....36 g

Conch Salad

Preparation time: 10 min ✦ Serves 4 ✦ Serving size: 1/4 recipe

1 lb fresh or frozen conch, diced into small pieces
1 medium onion, diced
1 medium bell pepper, diced
1 14.5-oz can diced tomatoes
2 medium fresh tomatoes, diced
1 cup lemon juice
1/2 cup orange juice
1/2 tsp salt
Black pepper and hot sauce to taste

Mix all ingredients together. Add black pepper and hot sauce to taste.
Chill, then serve.

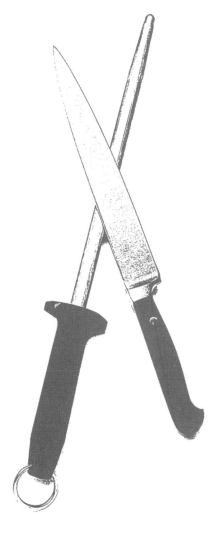

Exchanges
1 Starch
1/2 Fruit
2 Very Lean Meat

Calories..........................172
  Calories from Fat........... 13
Total Fat .... 1 g
  Saturated Fat............... 0.3 g
  Trans Fat .... 0 g
Cholesterol .... 44 mg
Sodium..........................327 mg
Total Carbohydrate ..... 21 g
  Dietary Fiber .... 3 g
  Sugars .... 12 g
Protein .... 21 g

Creole Red Snapper

Preparation time: 20 min ✦ Serves 4 ✦ Serving size: 1 fillet

Nonstick cooking spray
1/4 cup frozen chopped onion
1/4 cup frozen chopped green pepper
1 tsp minced garlic
1 14.5-oz can diced tomatoes, undrained
2 tsp Worcestershire sauce
2 tsp red wine vinegar
1/2 tsp basil
4 red snapper fillets (4 oz each)

1 Spray a large skillet with nonstick cooking spray and heat over medium-high heat until hot. Add onion, green pepper, and garlic; sauté until tender, stirring frequently.

2 Add tomatoes with juice, Worcestershire sauce, vinegar, and basil. Bring to a boil. Add fish fillets, spooning tomato mixture over the fish to make sure each fillet is coated.

3 Reduce heat and simmer, covered, for 10–12 minutes or until the fish flakes easily with a fork.

Exchanges
1 Vegetable
3 Very Lean Meat

Calories........................141
    Calories from Fat.......... 15
Total Fat ....2 g
    Saturated Fat............... 0.3 g
    Trans Fat .... 0 g
Cholesterol .... 41 mg
Sodium........................ 289 mg
Total Carbohydrate....... 6 g
    Dietary Fiber .... 1 g
    Sugars .... 5 g
Protein .... 24 g

Curried Grouper Steaks

Preparation time: 20 min ✦ Serves 4 ✦ Serving size: 1 steak

- 4 grouper steaks
- 1/4 tsp salt
- 1/2 tsp pepper
- 4 Tbsp curry powder
- 1 cup flour
- 2 Tbsp canola oil
- 1 Tbsp garlic powder
- 1 cup sliced unpeeled apples
- 1 cup orange juice

Season the fish with salt and pepper. In a mixing bowl, combine 2 Tbsp curry powder and the flour. Dredge the grouper in the flour and shake off any excess. Heat the oil in a large frying pan; then add the fish and cook for 3–4 minutes over high heat. Turn each steak and cook for 2 more minutes. Remove the fish and place on serving plate. To the skillet, add the garlic powder, apples, orange juice, and remaining 2 Tbsp curry powder. Simmer until liquid is reduced. Pour the sauce over the fish and serve.

Exchanges
2 Carbohydrate
3 Lean Meat

Calories 317
 Calories from Fat 82
Total Fat .... 9 g
 Saturated Fat .... 0.9 g
 Trans Fat .... 0 g
Cholesterol .... 52 mg
Sodium .... 209 mg
Total Carbohydrate ..... 28 g
 Dietary Fiber .... 3 g
 Sugars .... 11 g
Protein .... 31 g

Curry Chicken Sandwich

Preparation time: 15 min ✦ Serves 6 ✦ Serving size: 3 oz

2 1/2 cups cooked light and dark chicken meat, cubed
1/2 cup chopped nuts, such as walnuts
1/2 cup celery, chopped
2 Tbsp onion, finely chopped
1/2 cup fat-free mayonnaise
2 Tbsp fat-free sour cream
1 tsp curry powder
1/8 tsp Cajun seasoning

In a food processor, process the chicken until it's finely chopped. Transfer to a large bowl. Add the nuts, celery, and onion and stir well. In a separate bowl, combine the mayonnaise, sour cream, curry powder, and Cajun seasoning. Pour over the chicken mixture and stir well. Refrigerate. Spread over a small bun and add lots of lettuce.

Exchanges
1/2 Carbohydrate
2 Lean Meat
1 Fat

Calories..........................196
   Calories from Fat........... 97
Total Fat ....11 g
   Saturated Fat................ 1.9 g
   Trans Fat .... 0 g
Cholesterol .... 52 mg
Sodium......................... 205 mg
Total Carbohydrate .... 5 g
   Dietary Fiber .... 1 g
   Sugars .... 2 g
Protein .... 19 g

Dan the Man's Pork Tenderloin

Preparation time: 15 min ✦ Serves 8 ✦ Serving size: 3 oz

2	lb pork tenderloin, unseasoned
1/2	cup lite soy sauce
1	Tbsp jerk seasoning
1/4	cup bourbon
1/4	cup Splenda® Brown Sugar Blend
1	10-oz bag baby spinach
	Nonstick cooking spray
1/4	tsp kosher salt
2	tsp minced garlic

1 Marinate the pork tenderloin in the soy sauce and jerk seasoning for 2 hours.

2 Combine the bourbon and Splenda® in separate bowl.

3 Brush the bourbon and Splenda® mixture over the tenderloin while grilling. Cook until tenderloin reaches 155°F internal temperature.

4 Grease a sauté pan with nonstick cooking spray. Sauté the spinach, salt, and garlic over high heat for 3 minutes, until slightly wilted. Toss frequently and remove from heat. Spread the spinach in serving dish. Layer the sliced tenderloin on a bed of spinach.

Exchanges
1/2 Carbohydrate
4 Very Lean Meat

Calories	193
Calories from Fat	37
Total Fat	4 g
Saturated Fat	1.4 g
Trans Fat	0 g
Cholesterol	66 mg
Sodium	638 mg
Total Carbohydrate	9 g
Dietary Fiber	1 g
Sugars	7 g
Protein	25 g

Derek's Catfish Fry

Preparation time: 10 min ✦ Serves 8 ✦ Serving size: 3 oz

8	3.5-oz catfish fillets
2	cups nonfat milk
2	cups yellow cornmeal
2	tsp seasoned salt
2	tsp pepper
1/2	tsp onion powder
1/2	tsp garlic powder
	Nonstick cooking spray
8	lemon wedges

1 Place the catfish fillets in a single layer in a shallow dish. Cover with milk.

2 Combine the cornmeal and the salt, pepper, onion powder, and garlic powder in a shallow dish.

3 Remove the catfish fillets from the milk, allowing excess to drip off. Dredge the catfish fillets in the cornmeal mixture, shaking off excess.

4 To oven fry the fish, lightly spray each fillet with nonstick cooking spray. Bake at 400°F for 15 minutes. Serve with lemon wedges.

Exchanges
1 Starch
2 Lean Meat
1/2 Fat

Calories 212
　　Calories from Fat........... 67
Total Fat .... 7　g
　　Saturated Fat............... 1.7　g
　　Trans Fat .... 0　g
Cholesterol .... 58　mg
Sodium ....277　mg
Total Carbohydrate ......16　g
　　Dietary Fiber .... 1　g
　　Sugars .... 2　g
Protein .... 19　g

Ernestine's Beef Pie

Preparation time: 20 min ✦ Serves 12 ✦ Serving size: 1/2 cup

1	8.5-oz corn bread mix
1	lb very lean ground beef (85% lean, 15% fat)
1	large onion, chopped
1	cup bell pepper, chopped
1	16-oz can dark kidney beans, rinsed and drained
1	15.25-oz can whole kernel corn, drained
2	cups tomato sauce
1	14-oz can low-sodium diced tomatoes, undrained
1	4-oz can chopped green chilies
3	tsp chili powder
1 1/2	tsp ground cumin
3/4	tsp garlic powder

1 Prepare the corn bread mix according to the package instructions (usually requires an egg and some nonfat milk), but do not bake. Set aside.

2 In a large skillet over medium heat, brown the beef until done. Drain away any fat in the skillet. Add the onion and bell pepper. Add all remaining ingredients and bring to a boil. Stir often. Reduce heat and simmer for 10 minutes.

3 Transfer the meat mixture to a large casserole dish. Spread out evenly. Pour the uncooked corn bread batter over the meat. Bake at 400°F for 20 minutes or until corn bread is done.

Exchanges
1 1/2 Starch
1 Vegetable
1 Lean Meat
1/2 Fat

Calories	213
Calories from Fat	56
Total Fat	6 g
Saturated Fat	2.4 g
Trans Fat	0.3 g
Cholesterol	40 mg
Sodium	591 mg
Total Carbohydrate	32 g
Dietary Fiber	5 g
Sugars	10 g
Protein	13 g

Eunice's Bourbon Cornish Hens

Preparation time: 20 min ✦ Serves 4 ✦ Serving size: 1/2 Cornish hen

> 2 lbs Cornish hen (about 2 whole hens), skin removed
> Salt and black pepper, to taste
> 3 cups reduced-sodium, low-fat chicken broth
> 3 Tbsp shallots, minced
> 2 Tbsp bourbon
> 4 limes, juiced
> 1/8 cup Splenda® Brown Sugar Blend
> 2 cups crushed pineapples, in juice
> 2 Tbsp light, soft, tub margarine

1 Rinse and split the hens down the middle for baking. Season each with salt and pepper to taste and bake at 375°F for 1 hour. Baste the hens with 2 cups chicken broth.

2 Use the hen drippings to sauté the shallots for a few minutes. Add bourbon and flame. Add the lime juice, Splenda®, and crushed pineapple. Cook until sauce reduces. Add the remaining 1 cup chicken broth and reduce again. Stir in the margarine and remove from heat. Pour sauce over Cornish hens. Serve hot.

Exchanges
1 Starch
1/2 Carbohydrate
3 Very Lean Meat
1 Fat

Calories 267
   Calories from Fat.......... 63
Total Fat .... 7 g
   Saturated Fat............... 1.4 g
   Trans Fat .... 0 g
Cholesterol .... 98 mg
Sodium ....193 mg
Total Carbohydrate ...... 25 g
   Dietary Fiber .... 1 g
   Sugars .... 22 g
Protein .... 24 g

Freshwater Sweetness with Mango Salsa

Preparation time: 15 min ✦ Serves 4 ✦ Serving size: 1/2 fillet

Mango salsa

2 small ripe mangoes, chopped
1 Tbsp grated orange rind
1/2 cup chopped red, green, yellow bell peppers
1/2 cup chopped red onion
1 tsp fresh grated ginger
1 Tbsp fresh chopped cilantro
3 lemons (juiced)

Fish

2 6-oz catfish fillets
1 tsp Scotch bonnet pepper sauce
1 tsp seasoned salt
1 tsp lemon pepper
2 Tbsp olive oil

1 Prepare the mango salsa. Mix all of the ingredients and let stand for 4 hours.

2 Prepare the catfish by rubbing it with the spices and oil. Marinate for 30 minutes.

3 Sauté the fish in a thin layer of olive oil. Cook for 4–8 minutes on each side. Serve with mango salsa on top.

Exchanges
1 1/2 Fruit
2 Lean Meat
1 1/2 Fat

Calories........................270
　Calories from Fat..........121
Total Fat .... 13　g
　Saturated Fat.................. 2　g
　Trans Fat .... 0　g
Cholesterol .... 49　mg
Sodium.........................551　mg
Total Carbohydrate ..... 24　g
　Dietary Fiber .... 3　g
　Sugars ....18　g
Protein ....16　g

Glazed Pork Chops

Preparation time: 20 min ✦ Serves 4 ✦ Serving size: 1 pork chop

>   3/4   cup apricot preserves, no sugar added
>   1/4   cup fat-free Italian salad dressing
>   2 1/2   Tbsp Dijon-style mustard
>   4   pork chops (1 1/2 lb each)

1 Prepare a marinade by using a blender to combine the apricot preserves, Italian dressing, and mustard.

2 Place the pork chops in zip-top plastic bag. Reserve 1/4 cup of marinade and refrigerate. Pour the rest over the pork chops. Place in the refrigerator for about 3 hours or overnight.

3 Remove the pork chops and discard the marinade. Bake at 425°F for 45 minutes, turning, and brush with the reserved marinade while cooking. Cook until pork chops are done.

Exchanges
1/2 Carbohydrate
3 Lean Meat

Calories	192	
Calories from Fat	64	
Total Fat	7	g
Saturated Fat	2.6	g
Trans Fat	0	g
Cholesterol	71	mg
Sodium	242	mg
Total Carbohydrate	5	g
Dietary Fiber	0	g
Sugars	1	g
Protein	25	g

Grilled Salmon

Preparation time: 10 min ✦ Serves 6 ✦ Serving size: 1 fillet

- 1/2   cup balsamic vinegar
- 2   Tbsp Splenda® Brown Sugar Blend
- 1   tsp sesame oil
- 1   tsp fresh ginger
- 4   green onions, diced
- 6   4-oz salmon fillets

Mix the first five ingredients together and brush over the salmon fillets. Grill until the fish is firm.

Exchanges
1/2 Carbohydrate
3 Lean Meat
1/2 Fat

Calories...................... 232
    Calories from Fat........... 94
Total Fat .... 10 g
    Saturated Fat............... 1.8 g
    Trans Fat .... 0 g
Cholesterol .... 77 mg
Sodium.......................... 62 mg
Total Carbohydrate .... 9 g
    Dietary Fiber .... 0 g
    Sugars .... 7 g
Protein .... 24 g

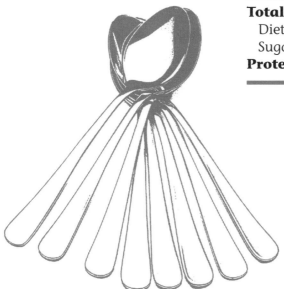

Jay's Chicken Chili

Preparation time: 20 min ✦ Serves 8 ✦ Serving size: 1 cup

1	Tbsp olive oil
1 1/2	lb chicken breast, skin removed, chopped
1	cup onion, chopped
1 1/2	cups reduced-sodium, low-fat chicken broth
1/2	cup chili peppers
1	tsp garlic powder
1	tsp cumin
1/2	tsp oregano
1/2	tsp coriander
	Dash red pepper
2	14.5-oz cans navy beans, drained and rinsed
3	scallions, chopped
1/2	cup Monterey jack cheese
1	cup chopped tomatoes
	Garnish: jalapeño peppers

Heat the oil in a large pot. Add the chicken and onion, and sauté for 4–5 minutes. Add the chicken broth, chili peppers, garlic powder, cumin, oregano, coriander, and red pepper. Bring to a boil. Reduce heat and simmer for 15 minutes. Stir in the beans; simmer for 10 minutes. Serve topped with scallions, cheese, chopped tomatoes, and jalapeño peppers.

Exchanges
1 Starch
1 Vegetable
3 Very Lean Meat
1 Fat

Calories	265	
Calories from Fat	61	
Total Fat	7	g
Saturated Fat	2.2	g
Trans Fat	0	g
Cholesterol	56	mg
Sodium	257	mg
Total Carbohydrate	24	g
Dietary Fiber	5	g
Sugars	4	g
Protein	27	g

Jeanette's Praline Chicken

Preparation time: 15 min ✦ Serves 6 ✦ Serving size: 1/2 breast

6	split chicken breasts, skinned and boneless
2	tsp salt and pepper combined
1 1/2	Tbsp canola oil
1/2	cup maple syrup
2	Tbsp brown sugar
1/3	cup water
1/3	cup chopped pecans

Season the chicken with the salt and pepper combination. Heat the oil in a hot skillet. Brown the chicken on both sides until done. Remove from heat and place on platter. Pour the syrup and brown sugar into the skillet with the drippings. Mix well. Add water and pecans, and stir until heated. Let sauce reduce until thickened. Spoon sauce over chicken. Serve hot.

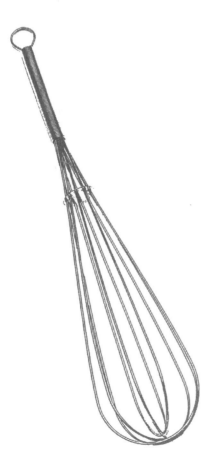

Exchanges
1 Carbohydrate
3 Very Lean Meat
1 1/2 Fat

Calories	254	
Calories from Fat	97	
Total Fat	11	g
Saturated Fat	1.4	g
Trans Fat	0	g
Cholesterol	66	mg
Sodium	254	mg
Total Carbohydrate	14	g
Dietary Fiber	1	g
Sugars	13	g
Protein	25	g

Mamma Mia, Chicken Scaloppini

Preparation time: 20 min ✦ Serves 6 ✦ Serving size: 3 oz

> 1 lb chicken or turkey breast, sliced very thin into 12 slices, skin removed
> Salt and freshly ground black pepper, to taste
> 2 Tbsp light, soft, tub margarine
> 1 lb mushrooms, sliced
> 2 large shallots, finely chopped
> 3/4 cup dry white wine
> 1 cup 100% fat-free, reduced-sodium chicken broth
> 1/4 tsp saffron threads
> 3/4 cup fat-free half and half
> 1/2 cup frozen peas, thawed
> Capers

1 Sprinkle the poultry with salt and pepper. Melt 1 Tbsp margarine in a heavy large frying pan over high heat. Working in batches, add the meat and sauté until just cooked through and golden, about 45–60 seconds per side. Transfer the poultry to a platter.

2 Melt 1 Tbsp of the remaining margarine in the same pan over high heat. Add the mushrooms and shallots. Sprinkle with salt and pepper, and sauté until the mushrooms are golden brown, about 8 minutes. Add the wine, broth, and saffron; simmer until the liquid is reduced by half, about 5 minutes. Add the half and half and boil until the sauce thickens slightly, stirring often, about 4 minutes. Add the peas and return the sauce to a simmer. Season the sauce, to taste, with salt and pepper. Throw in a few capers for flavor. To serve, place two slices of meat on a plate and lightly cover with sauce.

Exchanges
1/2 Carbohydrate
3 Very Lean Meat
1/2 Fat

Calories 167
    Calories from Fat 40
Total Fat .... 4 g
    Saturated Fat .... 0.9 g
    Trans Fat .... 0 g
Cholesterol .... 46 mg
Sodium .... 206 mg
Total Carbohydrate ..... 10 g
    Dietary Fiber .... 2 g
    Sugars .... 4 g
Protein .... 20 g

Orange Ginger Cornish Hens

Preparation time: 20 min ✦ Serves 12 ✦ Serving size: 1/2 Cornish hen

4	cloves garlic, minced
1/4	cup chipped ginger
1/2	cup lite soy sauce
1/2	cup orange juice
1/2	cup Splenda® No Calorie Sweetener
6	Cornish hens (about 1 lb each), skin removed
1	lemon, quartered
1	orange, quartered

Blend the garlic, ginger, soy sauce, and orange juice together in a food processor to make a marinade. Reserve half and refrigerate. Pour the other half over the hens, and marinate in the refrigerator overnight. Bake for 1 hour in oven at 350°F. Baste with reserved marinade every 15 minutes. Remove the citrus from the core when hens are done. If desired, you can grill the hens and baste every 15 minutes until done.

Exchanges
3 Very Lean Meat

Calories........................130
    Calories from Fat...........31
Total Fat .... 3 g
    Saturated Fat............... 0.9 g
    Trans Fat .... 0 g
Cholesterol .... 95 mg
Sodium........................ 247 mg
Total Carbohydrate .... 2 g
    Dietary Fiber .... 0 g
    Sugars .... 1 g
Protein .... 22 g

Oriental Pork Loin

Preparation time: 15 min ✦ Serves 5 ✦ Serving size: 3 oz

1	Tbsp Chinese five spice
	(find this in the Asian foods aisle of your grocery store)
2	Tbsp sesame oil
1/2	tsp salt
1 1/2	tsp garlic powder
1	tsp crushed red pepper
1	tsp dark brown sugar
5	1/3-inch-thick pork tenderloins

Combine the first six ingredients in a small bowl. Stir and form a paste. Rub the paste on both sides of each pork loin. Grill the pork loin over medium heat. Cook until pork is 160°F. Let the meat rest for 5 minutes before serving.

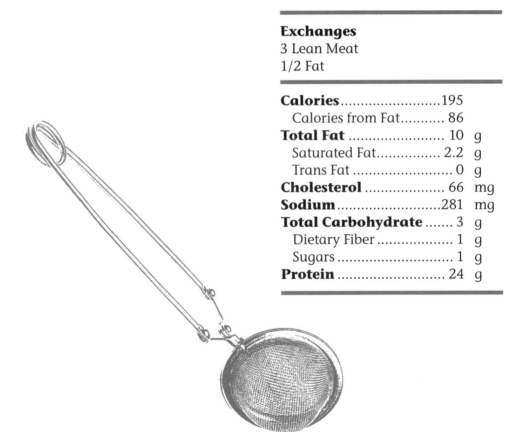

Exchanges
3 Lean Meat
1/2 Fat

Calories	195	
Calories from Fat	86	
Total Fat	10	g
Saturated Fat	2.2	g
Trans Fat	0	g
Cholesterol	66	mg
Sodium	281	mg
Total Carbohydrate	3	g
Dietary Fiber	1	g
Sugars	1	g
Protein	24	g

Pesto Fish

Preparation time: 20 min ✦ Serves 6 ✦ Serving size: 1/2 cup

1/4	cup tightly packed fresh basil leaves
3	Tbsp fat-free Italian dressing
1	garlic clove, minced
1/4	tsp salt
1/8	tsp black pepper
1 1/2	lb flounder or any type of white fish

Combine the basil, Italian dressing, garlic, salt, and pepper in a blender or food processor. Blend until finely chopped. Season the fish fillets with salt and pepper. Arrange the fillets in a baking dish and spread the basil mixture on top. Place the dish on a baking rack 6 inches under broiler for 4–5 minutes or until the fish is firm and opaque and flakes easily with a fork.

Exchanges
3 Very Lean Meat

Calories........................108
   Calories from Fat.......... 12
Total Fat .... 1 g
   Saturated Fat............... 0.3 g
   Trans Fat .... 0 g
Cholesterol .... 60 mg
Sodium.........................267 mg
Total Carbohydrate .... 1 g
   Dietary Fiber .... 0 g
   Sugars .... 1 g
Protein .... 21 g

Pit-Master Weaver's Grilled Guava Barbeque Pork Loin

Preparation time: 25 min ✦ Serves 10 ✦ Serving size: 3 oz

1	cup guava paste (find this in the Hispanic foods section of your grocery store)
2 1/2	lb large boneless pork loin
1	Tbsp Creole seasoning spice or jerk rub
12	oz barbeque sauce
1	lemon, juiced

1 Preheat the grill.

2 Melt the guava paste on a stove. Add a little bit of water to soften it up. Cook until soft; then strain and let cool. Season the pork loin with 2 tsp Creole seasoning or jerk rub.

3 To make the sauce, in medium pot over medium heat, add the barbeque sauce with 1 tsp Creole seasoning or jerk rub. Add the guava puree and lemon juice. Mix well; then cook on the stove for 10 minutes. Put the pork loin on the grill. Brush the loin with the sauce and grill for 10 minutes. Baste loin again and turn over. Baste this side as well and grill for 15 minutes. Continue to baste and turn until desired doneness is reached. Once the meat is cooled, slice very thin and serve with rolls.

Exchanges
2 Carbohydrate
2 Lean Meat

Calories	263
Calories from Fat	70
Total Fat	8 g
Saturated Fat	2.6 g
Trans Fat	0 g
Cholesterol	59 mg
Sodium	492 mg
Total Carbohydrate	27 g
Dietary Fiber	1 g
Sugars	23 g
Protein	21 g

Roniece's Crawfish Étouffée

Preparation time: 20 min ✦ Serves 12 ✦ Serving size: 1/3 cup étouffée and 1/2 cup rice

1	cup flour
2	Tbsp canola oil
2	cups onions, chopped
1	cup bell pepper, chopped
2	cups celery, chopped
2	cups water
2	shrimp or fish bouillon cubes
2	Tbsp garlic, minced
1	tsp oregano
1	tsp thyme
2–3	bay leaves
1	lb crawfish, frozen and without shells

1 Heat the oven to 400°F and brown the flour without oil. Stir often, until the flour turns the color of peanut butter. Watch carefully until brown. Place in a glass jar once cooled. Save any unused portions.

2 In large cast iron skillet, heat the oil. Sauté the vegetables until tender for 8 minutes. Add the browned flour and mix well. Add the 2 cups water, bouillon cubes, garlic, oregano, thyme, and bay leaves. Bring to a boil and simmer. If the sauce is too thick, add more water. Add frozen crawfish and simmer. Reduce heat. Simmer for 30 minutes and remove from heat. Serve in a martini glass with 1 oz of rice for appetizer or serve in a soup bowl with 2 oz of rice. Garnish with a single piece of shrimp on the lip of the glass. (Nutritional analysis applies to the entrée, not the appetizer serving.)

This is a new way to make a roux without any oil, and it can be prepared days ahead of time. This can be done ahead because it takes time to brown the flour. Any unused flour can be saved for future sauces, or gravies.

Exchanges
1 1/2 Starch
1 Vegetable
1 Very Lean Meat
1/2 Fat

Calories..........................191
Calories from Fat........... 28
Total Fat .... 3 g
Saturated Fat............... 0.4 g
Trans Fat .... 0 g
Cholesterol .... 48 mg
Sodium......................... 230 mg
Total Carbohydrate ......31 g
Dietary Fiber .... 1 g
Sugars .... 2 g
Protein .... 10 g

Rojean's Award-Winning Sea Bass with Pistachio Crust

Preparation time: 15 min ✦ Serves 2 ✦ Serving size: 1 fillet

2	4-oz fillets Chilean sea bass
1	Tbsp olive oil
	Lemon pepper to taste
	Old Bay Seasoning to taste
1/4	cup lemon juice
1/2	cup crushed unsalted pistachios
1/4	cup plain bread crumbs

Rub the fish with the olive oil. Gently season the fish with lemon pepper and/or Old Bay Seasoning, to taste. Lay the fillets on a baking sheet or casserole. In a separate bowl, mix together the lemon juice, pistachios, and bread crumbs. Spread this mixture over the tops of each fish fillet. Bake or broil for 20 minutes, until the fish flakes easily with a fork.

Exchanges
1 1/2 Carbohydrate
4 Lean Meat
2 Fat

Calories	404	
Calories from Fat	215	
Total Fat	24	g
Saturated Fat	2.8	g
Trans Fat	0	g
Cholesterol	47	mg
Sodium	185	mg
Total Carbohydrate	20	g
Dietary Fiber	4	g
Sugars	4	g
Protein	29	g

Seafood Mix

Preparation time: 20 min ✦ Serves 6 ✦ Serving size: 1/6 recipe

1	Tbsp canola oil
1	28-oz can tomatoes, drained and chopped
2	Tbsp tomato paste
2	Tbsp chopped parsley
2	cloves garlic, smashed and chopped
1	cup onions, chopped
1/2	cup crabmeat, well drained
1/2	lb scallops
1/2	lb shrimp, peeled and deveined
	Salt and pepper to taste
2	Tbsp garlic powder
1/2	cup shredded reduced-fat cheddar cheese

1 Heat the oil in a large frying pan. Add tomatoes, tomato paste, parsley, garlic, and onions. Cook until onions are soft. Add crabmeat, scallops, and shrimp; season with salt, pepper, and garlic powder. Cook for 3–4 minutes over medium-low heat.

2 Pour mixture into a large ovenproof dish. Sprinkle with cheese and broil until golden brown.

Exchanges
2 Vegetables
2 Lean Meat

Calories........................ 152
   Calories from Fat........... 48
Total Fat .... 5 g
   Saturated Fat................ 1.5 g
   Trans Fat .... 0 g
Cholesterol ....76 mg
Sodium.........................337 mg
Total Carbohydrate .... 9 g
   Dietary Fiber .... 2 g
   Sugars .... 4 g
Protein ....17 g

Seafood Pasta

Preparation time: 20 min ✦ Serves 6 ✦ Serving size 1/6 recipe

- 1   16-oz pkg spaghetti or angel hair pasta
- 1   16-oz jar marinara sauce
- 1/2 lb fish, scallops, or shrimp
  Freshly grated Parmesan cheese (*optional*)

Prepare the pasta according to package directions; drain. In a separate pan, heat the marinara sauce until warm. Add the seafood and cook for 10 minutes. Add the cooked pasta to the sauce; stir until blended. Top with grated cheese, if desired.

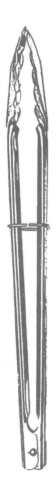

Exchanges
4 Starch
1 Vegetable
1 Very Lean Meat

Calories..........................373
   Calories from Fat........... 42
Total Fat .... 5 g
   Saturated Fat............... 0.8 g
   Trans Fat .... 0 g
Cholesterol .... 29 mg
Sodium......................... 364 mg
Total Carbohydrate ..... 64 g
   Dietary Fiber .... 6 g
   Sugars .... 6 g
Protein ....18 g

Seafood with Pineapple Glaze

Preparation time: 20 min ✦ Serves 8 ✦ Serving size: 1 fillet

2	Tbsp Splenda® Sugar Blend for Baking
2	Tbsp pineapple tidbits
1	Tbsp pineapple juice
1 1/4	tsp minced ginger
1	Tbsp garlic, minced
2	Tbsp rice vinegar
1	Tbsp fresh basil, chopped
1	dash red pepper
8	3-oz fish fillets, such as snapper
1/2	tsp salt
1/2	tsp black pepper
1	tsp canola oil

In a medium saucepan, combine the Splenda®, pineapple, pineapple juice, ginger, and garlic. Bring to a boil over high heat. Reduce heat and simmer for 3 minutes. Stir in the vinegar, basil, and red pepper. Sprinkle the fish fillets with salt and pepper. Heat the oil in a nonstick skillet over medium-high heat. Add fish and cook 2 minutes. Turn fish over. Spoon pineapple glaze evenly over fish. Transfer glazed fish to the oven and broil 4 minutes, until fish flakes with a fork.

Exchanges
1/2 Carbohydrate
2 Very Lean Meat

Calories	107	
Calories from Fat	15	
Total Fat	2	g
Saturated Fat	0.3	g
Trans Fat	0	g
Cholesterol	31	mg
Sodium	183	mg
Total Carbohydrate	4	g
Dietary Fiber	0	g
Sugars	4	g
Protein	18	g

Shrimp on Flats

Preparation time: 20 min ✦ Serves 4 ✦ Serving size: 1/4 recipe

12 oz uncooked large shrimp, peeled and deveined
5 tsp extra-virgin olive oil
1/4 tsp salt
1 tsp freshly ground black pepper
3 tsp fresh lime juice
1/4 cup lightly packed fresh Italian parsley leaves
1/4 cup fat-free sour cream
1/4 cup low-fat plain yogurt
3 Tbsp chopped fresh chives
1/4 cup finely chopped fresh tarragon or
1 Tbsp finely chopped fresh thyme leaves
2 Tbsp capers, drained
Flatbread

1 In a large bowl, toss the shrimp with 3 tsp (1 Tbsp) olive oil to coat. Sprinkle with salt and pepper. Heat a heavy large nonstick skillet over medium-high heat. Sauté the shrimp until they are just cooked through or pink, about 1 1/2 minutes per side. Transfer the shrimp to a plate and toss with 1 tsp lime juice. Cool completely. Cut the shrimp into small cubes.

2 Blend the parsley, sour cream, yogurt, and remaining 2 tsp lime juice in a food processor until the parsley is finely chopped. Season the sauce, to taste, with salt and pepper. Set the parsley sauce aside.

3 In a large bowl, toss the cooked shrimp with the chives, tarragon or thyme, capers, and remaining 2 tsp of oil to coat. Season the salad, to taste, with salt and pepper. Drain and spoon about 1 Tbsp of the shrimp salad on top of a slice of flatbread. Toast gently in the oven. Remove from oven, drizzle the parsley sauce over the salad, cut into small serving pieces, and serve immediately.

Exchanges
1 Starch
2 Very Lean Meat
1 1/2 Fat

Calories 217
 Calories from Fat 86
Total Fat .... 10 g
 Saturated Fat .... 1.4 g
 Trans Fat .... 0 g
Cholesterol .... 109 mg
Sodium .... 503 mg
Total Carbohydrate ......17 g
 Dietary Fiber .... 1 g
 Sugars .... 2 g
Protein .... 15 g

Spaghetti Supreme

Preparation time: 20 min ✦ Serves 15 ✦ Serving size: 1 cup

1	Tbsp olive oil
2	lb lean ground beef (85% lean, 15% fat)
4	large onions, chopped
2	large 28-oz cans tomatoes
1	Tbsp minced garlic
	Salt and pepper, to taste
1	tsp allspice
1	tsp cloves
3	bay leaves
1	12-oz can tomato paste
1	7-oz can mushrooms
1	lb spaghetti

1 In a large pot, heat the oil. Add the beef and onions, cooking until onions are translucent; drain away the fat. Add the tomatoes and two cans of water (just use the empty tomato cans, about 56 oz water), and let it come to a boil. Simmer for 2 hours. Add the garlic, salt, pepper, allspice, cloves, and bay leaves; simmer for 1 hour. Add tomato paste and mushrooms, cook for another 15 minutes.

2 Meanwhile, heat water in a large pot. Prepare the spaghetti according to the package instructions. Serve the sauce over hot pasta.

Exchanges
1 1/2 Starch
3 Vegetable
1 Medium-Fat Meat
1/2 Fat

Calories 295
　Calories from Fat 72
Total Fat .... 8 g
　Saturated Fat .... 2.5 g
　Trans Fat .... 0.4 g
Cholesterol .... 36 mg
Sodium .... 255 mg
Total Carbohydrate ..... 39 g
　Dietary Fiber .... 5 g
　Sugars .... 7 g
Protein ....18 g

Spinach Omelet

Preparation time: 15 min ✦ Serves 6 ✦ Serving size: 1 slice

3	cups egg substitute
1/2	cup fat-free feta cheese crumbled
1/4	cup freshly grated Parmesan cheese
1	tsp oregano
1/4	tsp thyme
	salt and pepper, to taste
1	Tbsp canola oil
2	tsp garlic
10	oz frozen leaf spinach, thawed, squeezed dry, and chopped

1 In large bowl, mix the egg substitute, cheeses, oregano, and thyme. Add salt and pepper to taste.

2 Heat the oil in a nonstick pan. Sauté the garlic in a large skillet, and add spinach until all moisture evaporates. Mix well. Add the egg and cheese mixture. Cook, but do not stir. Let the eggs cook around the edges for about 1 minute. Transfer the pan to the oven and bake at 350°F until the omelet has puffed and set, about 10–12 minutes. Slide the omelet onto a large plate, cut into wedges, and serve hot.

Variety Is the Spice of Life

You can be creative by adding

- Bell peppers
- Onions
- Mushrooms
- Zucchini

Exchanges
1 Vegetable
3 Very Lean Meat
1/2 Fat

Calories 139
   Calories from Fat........... 34
Total Fat .... 4 g
   Saturated Fat................ 0.9 g
   Trans Fat .... 0 g
Cholesterol .... 3 mg
Sodium .... 663 mg
Total Carbohydrate .... 5 g
   Dietary Fiber .... 1 g
   Sugars .... 2 g
Protein .... 21 g

Stuffed Chicken Breast with Crab

Preparation time: 20 min ✦ Serves 6 ✦ Serving size: 1/2 cup

2	Tbsp egg substitute
1/2	tsp salt
1/2	tsp pepper
1/?	tsp dry mustard
2	tsp Worcestershire sauce
1	Tbsp chopped fresh parsley
1	Tbsp fat-free mayonnaise (or soybean-based mayonnaise)
1/2	cup Maryland jumbo lump crab meat
6	4-oz raw chicken breasts, thinly sliced (as for scaloppini)

1 Preheat the oven to 350°F.

2 In a large bowl, combine the egg substitute, salt, pepper, mustard, Worcestershire sauce, parsley, and mayonnaise. Add the crab meat (be careful not to break up the lumps).

3 For each slice of chicken breast, take 1 Tbsp crabmeat mixture and place it just off center of the chicken cutlet. Roll the chicken around the crabmeat filling, so it looks like a chicken cigar. Be sure to start rolling from the edge of the meat closest to the crabmeat.

4 Place on a nonstick baking sheet, and bake for 12–15 minutes. Serve hot.

Exchanges
4 Very Lean Meat

Calories 147
    Calories from Fat 27
Total Fat .... 3 g
    Saturated Fat .... 0.8 g
    Trans Fat .... 0 g
Cholesterol .... 77 mg
Sodium .... 333 mg
Total Carbohydrate .... 1 g
    Dietary Fiber .... 0 g
    Sugars .... 1 g
Protein .... 27 g

Turkey Drumsticks

Preparation time: 20 min ✦ Serves 6 ✦ Serving size: 1 drumstick

        6 turkey drumsticks
        1 medium onion, sliced and separated into rings
        1 14.5-oz can stewed tomatoes
      1/2 cup boiling water
        2 tsp reduced-sodium, low-fat chicken bouillon granules
      1/2 tsp garlic
      1/2 tsp dried oregano
      1/2 tsp dried basil
        2 Tbsp minced fresh parsley

Place drumsticks in a 13 × 9 × 2-inch baking dish. Arrange the onion rings over the drumsticks. Pour tomatoes on top. Combine the water, bouillon, garlic, oregano, and basil; pour over onions and turkey. Sprinkle with parsley. Cover and bake at 325°F for 2 hours or until tender and a meat thermometer reads 180°F. Remove skin before serving.

Exchanges
1 Vegetable
4 Lean Meat

Calories..................... 246
    Calories from Fat............76
Total Fat .... 8 g
    Saturated Fat............... 2.8 g
    Trans Fat .... 0 g
Cholesterol .... 97 mg
Sodium........................ 355 mg
Total Carbohydrate .... 8 g
    Dietary Fiber .... 1 g
    Sugars .... 3 g
Protein .... 34 g

Vegetable-Rich Beef Stew

Preparation time: 20 min ✦ Serves 6 ✦ Serving size: 1/6 recipe

1	lb boneless beef sirloin tip roast, cut into 1-inch cubes
3	cups peeled potatoes, cubed
3	celery ribs, cut into 1-inch pieces
1 1/2	cup peeled sweet potatoes, cubed
3	large carrots, cut into 1-inch pieces
1	large onion, cut into 12 wedges
1	cup peeled rutabaga, cubed
1	Tbsp onion powder
2	tsp dried basil
1/2	tsp salt
1/4	tsp pepper
	Nonstick cooking spray
1/2	cup water
1	14.5-oz can stewed tomatoes

1 In a very large plastic zip-top bag, combine all of the ingredients except the water and tomatoes. Seal the bag; shake to coat evenly.

2 Transfer the mixture to a Dutch oven or 13 × 9 × 2-inch baking dish coated with nonstick cooking spray (the pan will be very full). Pour the water over the beef mixture. Cover and bake at 325°F for 1 1/2 hours. Stir in the tomatoes. Bake, uncovered, for 30–40 minutes, stirring after 25 minutes, or until beef and vegetables are tender.

Exchanges
1 1/2 Starch
3 Vegetable
1 Lean Meat
1/2 Fat

Calories 271
   Calories from Fat 43
Total Fat .... 5 g
   Saturated Fat .... 1.6 g
   Trans Fat .... 0 g
Cholesterol .... 44 mg
Sodium .... 460 mg
Total Carbohydrate ..... 40 g
   Dietary Fiber .... 5 g
   Sugars .... 11 g
Protein .... 19 g

Soul Food
Snacks

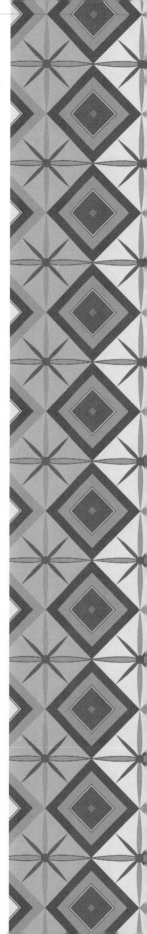

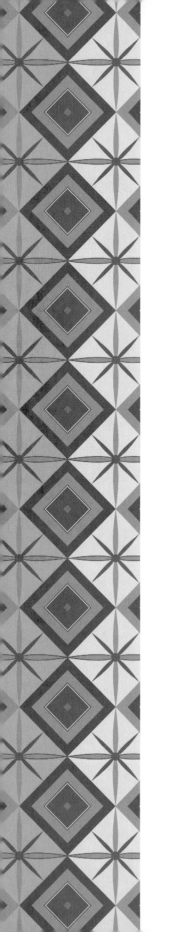

Bean Dip

Preparation time: 15 min ✦ Serves 8 ✦ Serving size: 1/8 recipe

1	16-oz can garbanzo beans
1/2	tsp lemon juice
1/2	tsp garlic powder
1	Tbsp canola oil
1/4	tsp lite soy sauce
1/8	tsp black pepper
1	Tbsp dried parsley flakes
1/3	cup water

Mash or blend all ingredients by hand or by using a food processor.
Refrigerate until ready to serve.

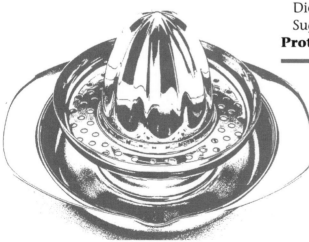

Exchanges
1 Starch

Calories 84
   Calories from Fat 21
Total Fat .... 2 g
   Saturated Fat .... 0.2 g
   Trans Fat .... 0 g
Cholesterol .... 0 mg
Sodium .... 177 mg
Total Carbohydrate ..... 13 g
   Dietary Fiber .... 3 g
   Sugars .... 2 g
Protein .... 3 g

Energy Bars

Preparation time: 15 min ✦ Serves 20 ✦ Serving size: 1 bar

        Nonstick cooking spray
1/3 cup unsalted margarine
1/2 cup canola oil
1/2 cup molasses
1/2 cup packed brown sugar
  1 cup unsweetened applesauce
  1 cup egg substitute
  1 cup wheat germ
  1 cup oatmeal, quick cooking
  2 tsp baking powder
  1 cup raisins
3/4 cup walnuts, finely chopped

Coat a 9 × 13-inch pan with nonstick cooking spray. Cream the margarine and oil until fluffy; beat in molasses, brown sugar, applesauce, and egg substitute. Combine the wheat germ, oatmeal, and baking powder; add to liquid mixture. Fold in raisins and walnuts. Spread mixture in the prepared pan and bake for 30 minutes at 350°F. Cut into bars and serve.

Exchanges
1 1/2 Carbohydrate
2 1/2 Fat

Calories.........................216
    Calories from Fat..........110
Total Fat .... 12 g
    Saturated Fat............... 1.3 g
    Trans Fat .... 0.5 g
Cholesterol .... 0 mg
Sodium........................... 66 mg
Total Carbohydrate ..... 24 g
    Dietary Fiber .... 2 g
    Sugars ....17 g
Protein .... 4 g

Nachos

Preparation time: 10 min ✦ Serves 12 ✦ Serving size: 1/12 recipe

> 1 13.5-oz bag baked tortilla chips
> 1 1/2 cups salsa
> 3/4 cup reduced-fat shredded cheese

Spread the chips on a baking sheet. Top each chip with 1 Tbsp salsa; then add a sprinkle of shredded cheese. Bake at 375°F until the cheese melts. Serve hot.

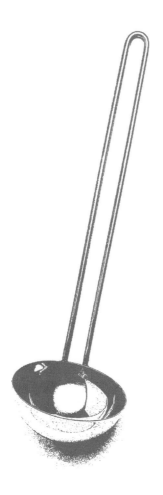

Exchanges
2 Starch

Calories	154	
Calories from Fat	24	
Total Fat	3	g
Saturated Fat	1.2	g
Trans Fat	0	g
Cholesterol	5	mg
Sodium	483	mg
Total Carbohydrate	30	g
Dietary Fiber	3	g
Sugars	1	g
Protein	6	g

Peach Tea

Preparation time: 10 min ✦ Serves 5 ✦ Serving size: 2 cups

        1/2 gallon water
        8–10 regular tea bags
          4 tsp Splenda® No Calorie Sweetener
          1 16-oz can peaches, packed in juice

Boil the water. Add tea bags. Remove the water from the heat and allow
the tea to steep. When the tea has cooled, pour it into a large pitcher and
sweeten to taste with Splenda®. Add canned peaches (and juice). Stir and
serve chilled.

Exchanges
1 Fruit

Calories.......................... 45
   Calories from Fat............. 0
Total Fat .... 0 g
   Saturated Fat.................. 0 g
   Trans Fat .... 0 g
Cholesterol .... 0 mg
Sodium...........................14 mg
Total Carbohydrate ..... 12 g
   Dietary Fiber .... 1 g
   Sugars .... 10 g
Protein .... 1 g

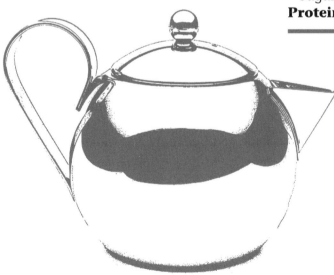

Peanut Butter Dip

Preparation time: 10 min ✦ Serves 20 ✦ Serving size: 1 Tbsp

> 1   cup creamy peanut butter
> 1/4 cup honey
> 1/2 tsp ground cinnamon

In a bowl, mix together the peanut butter, honey, and cinnamon. Continue mixing for about 5 minutes, until well mixed and smooth.

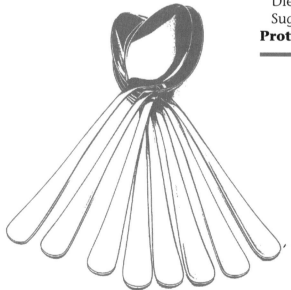

Exchanges
1/2 Carbohydrate
1 Fat

Calories........................... 90
   Calories from Fat...........61
Total Fat .... 7 g
   Saturated Fat............... 1.3 g
   Trans Fat .... 0 g
Cholesterol .... 0 mg
Sodium........................... 65 mg
Total Carbohydrate .... 6 g
   Dietary Fiber .... 1 g
   Sugars .... 4 g
Protein .... 3 g

Yogurt Fruit Dip

Preparation time: 10 min ✦ Serves 12 ✦ Serving size: 2 Tbsp

> 1 cup low-fat plain yogurt
> 1/2 cup diced peaches, packed in juice
> 1/2 cup unsweetened applesauce
> 2 Tbsp honey

Combine all ingredients in a bowl and stir until well blended. Refrigerate until chilled, and then serve. This dip can be used for dipping sliced fresh fruits.

Exchanges
1/2 Carbohydrate

Calories........................ 33
  Calories from Fat........... 3
Total Fat .... 0 g
  Saturated Fat................. 0 g
  Trans Fat .... 0 g
Cholesterol .... 1 mg
Sodium...........................18 mg
Total Carbohydrate .... 7 g
  Dietary Fiber .... 0 g
  Sugars .... 6 g
Protein .... 1 g

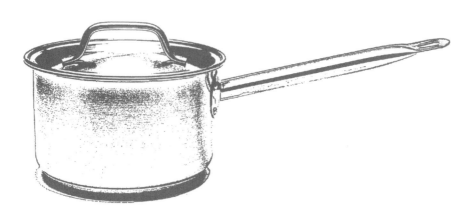

Soul Food
For Kids

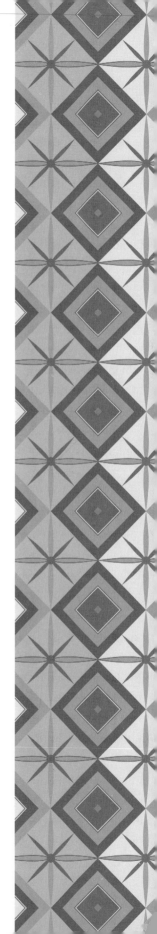

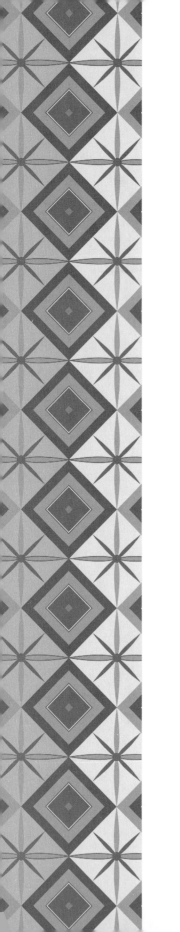

Apple Salad

Preparation time: 15 min ✦ Serves 6 ✦ Serving size: 1/6 recipe

3	medium apples (1 red, 1 yellow, and 1 green)
2	Tbsp lemon juice
1	stalk celery, sliced
1	cup seedless grapes, halved
1/2	cup golden raisins
1/4	cup chopped pecans
1/4	cup light mayonnaise
2	tsp Splenda® No Calorie Sweetener

1 Cut the apples into slices using an apple corer or slicer. Cut each slice into two or three pieces.

2 Place apples and lemon juice in a bowl and toss to coat with lemon juice.

3 Add celery, grapes, raisins, and pecans to apples. Toss to mix.

4 In a small bowl, whisk together the mayonnaise and Splenda®. Spoon onto salad and toss to coat.

5 Cover and refrigerate until serving time.

Exchanges
2 Fruit
1 Fat

Calories	159	
Calories from Fat	63	
Total Fat	7	g
Saturated Fat	0.9	g
Trans Fat	0	g
Cholesterol	3	mg
Sodium	97	mg
Total Carbohydrate	26	g
Dietary Fiber	3	g
Sugars	20	g
Protein	1	g

Banana Boat

Preparation time: 10 min ✦ Serves 4 ✦ Serving size: 1/2 banana

  2   medium bananas, with peel
20   miniature marshmallows
  2   Tbsp semisweet chocolate chips

Slit each banana lengthwise through the peel, making sure not to cut all
the way through to the other side. Stuff the bananas with marshmallows
and chocolate chips. Wrap each banana in aluminum foil and cook in a
300°F oven for 5 minutes or until chocolate is melted. Eat with a spoon.

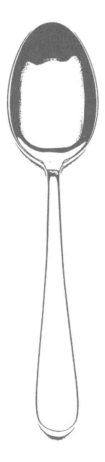

Exchanges
1 Fruit
1/2 Carbohydrate

Calories........................... 92
   Calories from Fat............16
Total Fat .... 2 g
   Saturated Fat.................. 1 g
   Trans Fat .... 0 g
Cholesterol .... 0 mg
Sodium............................. 3 mg
Total Carbohydrate ..... 21 g
   Dietary Fiber .... 2 g
   Sugars .... 13 g
Protein .... 1 g

Cereal Bars

Preparation time: 15 min ✦ Serves 30 ✦ Serving size: 1 square or ball

- 1/2 cup unsalted margarine
- 20 oz miniature marshmallows
- 12 cups all bran cereal

Melt the margarine slowly on the stovetop at medium heat. When margarine is melted, add the marshmallows. Remove from heat when all of the marshmallows are melted. Pour into a large bowl; mix with cereal and distribute evenly. Pour into a large baking pan and cut into 30 small squares or shape into small balls. Serve at room temperature.

Exchanges
2 Carbohydrate
1/2 Fat

Calories........................151
    Calories from Fat........... 34
Total Fat .... 4 g
    Saturated Fat............... 0.7 g
    Trans Fat .... 0.5 g
Cholesterol .... 0 mg
Sodium.......................... 73 mg
Total Carbohydrate ..... 34 g
    Dietary Fiber .... 8 g
    Sugars .... 20 g
Protein .... 3 g

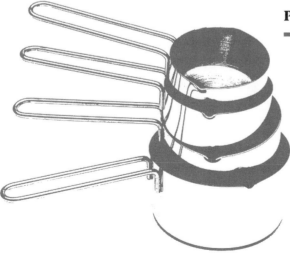

Cheese Ball

Preparation time: 10 min ✦ Serves 16 ✦ Serving size: 1/16 recipe

1	8-oz pkg fat-free cream cheese, softened
1	cup reduced-fat cheddar cheese, finely shredded
2	tsp Worcestershire sauce
1	tsp garlic powder
1/2	tsp fresh ground pepper
3/4	cup chopped walnuts
	Plastic wrap

Mix the cream cheese and cheddar cheese with an electric mixer on medium speed until well blended. Add the Worcestershire sauce, garlic powder, and pepper and mix well. Spoon into a bowl, cover with plastic wrap, and refrigerate for 1 hour. Remove from the refrigerator, form into a ball, and roll in the chopped walnuts to cover. Wrap cheese ball in plastic wrap and refrigerate for at least 3 hours. Place on serving plate and surround with crackers.

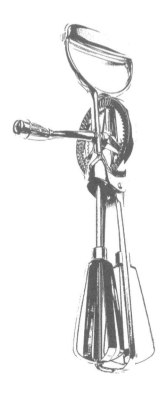

Exchanges
1 Lean Meat
1/2 Fat

Calories 73
   Calories from Fat 47
Total Fat .... 5 g
   Saturated Fat .... 1.2 g
   Trans Fat .... 0 g
Cholesterol .... 7 mg
Sodium .... 169 mg
Total Carbohydrate .... 2 g
   Dietary Fiber .... 0 g
   Sugars .... 1 g
Protein .... 5 g

Create-a-Portrait Meal

Preparation time: 15 min ✦ Serves 8 ✦ Serving size: 2 cups

Dipping sauce

1/2 cup light ranch or green goddess salad dressing

Assorted vegetables

2 cups baby carrots

2 cups grape tomatoes

1/2 cup raisins

2 cups broccoli florets

2 cups cauliflower florets

2 cups baby spinach

2 cups sliced cucumber, squash, or zucchini

1 cup red pepper strips

1 cup yellow pepper strips

1/2 cup fat-free croutons

1 cup tri-color pasta spirals, cooked

Create edible art or portraits with this variety of healthy vegetables. Allow your child's imagination to guide the way the meal looks. He or she can design trees, gardens, happy faces, and so forth, using the salad dressing to draw. Once the art work is done, it's time to eat and enjoy.

Exchanges

1/2 Starch
1/2 Fruit
2 Vegetable
1/2 Fat

Calories 145
   Calories from Fat........... 23
Total Fat .... 3 g
   Saturated Fat................ 0.4 g
   Trans Fat .... 0 g
Cholesterol .... 5 mg
Sodium .... 256 mg
Total Carbohydrate ..... 27 g
   Dietary Fiber .... 4 g
   Sugars .... 12 g
Protein .... 4 g

French Toast with Soul

Preparation time: 15 min ✦ Serves 3 ✦ Serving size: 2 French toast slices

3/4 cup nonfat milk
1/2 tsp vanilla
1 cup egg substitute
1 tsp cinnamon
1 tsp Splenda® No Calorie Sweetener
6 slices whole-wheat bread
Nonstick cooking spray

Mix the milk, vanilla, egg substitute, cinnamon, and Splenda® with a wire whisk. Dip the bread into the egg mixture, making sure both sides are covered. Lightly spray the griddle or skillet with nonstick cooking spray and preheat for a few seconds on medium heat. Using tongs, place the bread onto the griddle or skillet and cook until golden brown on both sides. Put two pieces of French toast on a serving plate. If desired, lightly top with margarine, fresh fruit, or sugar-free syrup (not included in nutritional analysis).

Exchanges
2 Starch
1 Very Lean Meat

Calories 187
   Calories from Fat 22
Total Fat .... 2 g
   Saturated Fat .... 0.6 g
   Trans Fat .... 0 g
Cholesterol .... 1 mg
Sodium .... 430 mg
Total Carbohydrate ..... 30 g
   Dietary Fiber .... 4 g
   Sugars .... 5 g
Protein .... 13 g

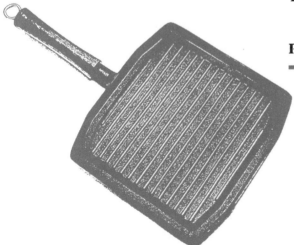

Grape Cow

Preparation time: 5 min ✦ Serves 2 ✦ Serving size: 1 cup

1/2 cup 100% grape juice
1/2 cup nonfat milk
1 cup sugar-free vanilla ice cream

Add the grape juice, milk, and ice cream to a blender. Blend on medium-high speed until smooth. Pour into glass and add straw.

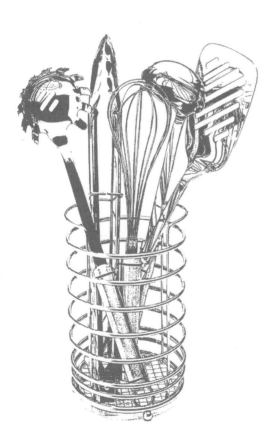

Exchanges
2 Carbohydrate

Calories 148
   Calories from Fat 22
Total Fat .... 2 g
   Saturated Fat .... 1.5 g
   Trans Fat .... 0 g
Cholesterol .... 6 mg
Sodium .... 102 mg
Total Carbohydrate ..... 27 g
   Dietary Fiber .... 0 g
   Sugars .... 16 g
Protein .... 5 g

New-Age Fruit Punch

Preparation time: 15 min ✦ Serves 24 ✦ Serving size: 6 oz

1	liter lemon-lime club soda
1/2	gallon canned pineapple juice
1	12-oz can frozen lime concentrate
2	medium bananas, sliced
2	medium oranges, sliced
1	16-oz bag frozen mixed fruit

Combine all of the ingredients in a punch bowl or large pitcher. Add more frozen fruit to keep it cool.

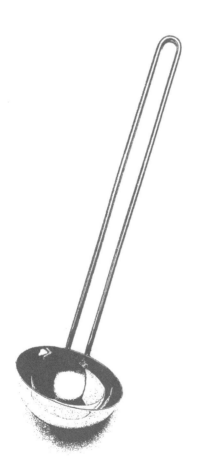

Exchanges
2 Fruit

Calories 105
   Calories from Fat 1
Total Fat .... 0 g
   Saturated Fat .... 0 g
   Trans Fat .... 0 g
Cholesterol .... 0 mg
Sodium .... 9 mg
Total Carbohydrate ..... 26 g
   Dietary Fiber .... 1 g
   Sugars .... 22 g
Protein .... 1 g

Parfait Cups

Preparation time: 15 min ✦ Serves 6 ✦ Serving size: 1 cup

> 1 cup fresh fruit (*select one from below*)
> —Fresh sliced strawberries
> —Blueberries
> —Blackberries
> —Raspberries
> —Bananas
> —Pineapple chunks
> 2 cups plain low-fat yogurt
> 1/2 cup low-fat granola cereal
> 2 Tbsp dry roasted almonds, chopped

Layer the fruit in a tall glass. Alternate a spoonful of fruit with a spoonful of plain low-fat yogurt. Top with granola and almonds.

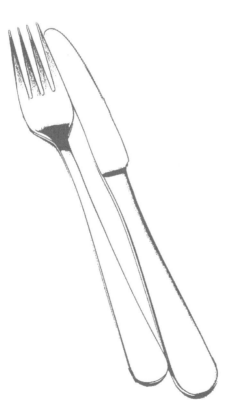

Exchanges
2 Fruit
1/2 Fat

Calories 143
    Calories from Fat........... 26
Total Fat .... 3 g
    Saturated Fat............... 0.6 g
    Trans Fat .... 0 g
Cholesterol .... 2 mg
Sodium .... 54 mg
Total Carbohydrate ..... 28 g
    Dietary Fiber .... 5 g
    Sugars .... 15 g
Protein .... 4 g

Pizza

Preparation time: 15 min ✦ Serves 8 ✦ Serving size: 1 slice

    1 8-oz pkg refrigerated reduced-fat crescent rolls
    1 8-oz pkg fat-free cream cheese, softened
    1 tsp dried oregano leaves
    1 tsp dried basil leaves
    1 tsp Italian seasoning
    1 tsp garlic powder
    2 Tbsp powdered buttermilk
    2 carrots, finely chopped
  1/2 cup chopped red bell peppers
  1/2 cup chopped green bell pepper
  1/2 cup fresh broccoli, chopped
  1/2 cup chopped green onions

1 Preheat oven to 375°F.

2 Roll out crescent rolls onto a large nonstick baking sheet. Stretch and flatten to form a single rectangular shape. Bake 11–13 minutes in the preheated oven or until golden brown. Allow to cool.

3 Place the cream cheese in a medium bowl. Mix the cream cheese with the oregano, basil, Italian seasoning, garlic powder, and powdered buttermilk. Spread the mixture over the cooled crust. Arrange the carrots, bell peppers, broccoli, and green onions on top. Chill in the refrigerator for approximately 1 hour. Cut into bite-size squares and serve.

Exchanges
1 Starch
1 Vegetable
1 Fat

Calories	154
Calories from Fat	43
Total Fat	5 g
Saturated Fat	1.1 g
Trans Fat	0 g
Cholesterol	5 mg
Sodium	454 mg
Total Carbohydrate	19 g
Dietary Fiber	2 g
Sugars	5 g
Protein	7 g

Pocket Pizza

Preparation time: 15 min ✦ Serves 8 ✦ Serving size: 1/2 pita pocket

4 whole-wheat pita pockets
8 1-oz slices reduced-fat mozzarella cheese
8 1-oz slices turkey breast
1/2 cup marinara (spaghetti) sauce

Cut each pita in half. Open each half to form a pocket. Stuff the inside of each half pita with 1 slice of cheese, 1 slice of turkey breast, and 1 Tbsp marinara sauce. Place pitas on a baking sheet, cover, and seal. Bake at 400°F for 10 minutes.

Exchanges
1 Starch
1 Lean Meat

Calories 140
   Calories from Fat 29
Total Fat .... 3 g
   Saturated Fat .... 1.3 g
   Trans Fat .... 0 g
Cholesterol .... 19 mg
Sodium .... 252 mg
Total Carbohydrate ...... 17 g
   Dietary Fiber .... 1 g
   Sugars .... 3 g
Protein .... 11 g

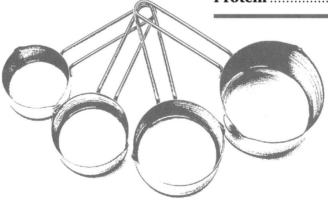

Snack Cups

Preparation time: 15 min ✦ Serves 4 ✦ Serving size: 1/4 recipe

4	whole bell peppers, use different colors: green, orange, red, and yellow
15	baby carrots
2	stalks of celery
8–10	asparagus spears
1	small jicama (about 1 lb)
1/2	cup reduced-fat ranch dressing

Take each pepper, cut off the top, and remove its seeds. Place the hollowed-out peppers upright on a platter. Pour the ranch dressing (or 1/2 cup nonfat fruit-flavored yogurt, if you prefer) into the hollowed-out peppers. Cut and slice all of the remaining vegetables into long strips.
Add some variety by making some of the strips longer than others.
Arrange the vegetable strips around the bell pepper cups and serve for a fun and tasty treat.

Exchanges
1/2 Carbohydrate
3 Vegetable
1 Fat

Calories 159
    Calories from Fat 41
Total Fat .... 5 g
    Saturated Fat .... 0.7 g
    Trans Fat .... 0 g
Cholesterol .... 10 mg
Sodium .... 398 mg
Total Carbohydrate ..... 26 g
    Dietary Fiber .... 9 g
    Sugars .... 8 g
Protein .... 4 g

Spinach Pizza

Preparation time: 15 min ✦ Serves 8 ✦ Serving size: 1 slice

2 Tbsp olive oil
1 Tbsp minced garlic
1 16-oz can crushed tomatoes, drained
   Prepared 12-inch pizza crust (such as Boboli brand)
   or low-carb flat bread
1 cup onions, chopped
8 oz spinach, chopped
1 cup sautéed mushrooms
1 cup minced green and red bell peppers
1 cup shredded fat-free cheddar cheese

Mix together the olive oil, garlic, and tomatoes, creating a marinara sauce; spread on top of pizza crust. Arrange the vegetables all over the crust, sprinkle cheese over pizza. Bake at 350°F for 7–10 minutes. Remove from heat once cheese melts. Cut into 8 slices and serve hot.

Exchanges
1 1/2 Starch
2 Vegetable
1 1/2 Fat

Calories 237
   Calories from Fat........... 65
Total Fat .... 7 g
   Saturated Fat................ 1.2 g
   Trans Fat .... 0 g
Cholesterol .... 1 mg
Sodium .... 600 mg
Total Carbohydrate ..... 32 g
   Dietary Fiber .... 3 g
   Sugars .... 6 g
Protein ....11 g

Strawberry Orange Spinach Salad

Preparation time: 15 min ✦ Serves 4 ✦ Serving size: 1/4 recipe

- 1   10-oz bag baby spinach
- 1   pint strawberries, rinsed and sliced
- 1   11-oz can mandarin oranges, drained
- 1/2   pint grape tomatoes
- 1/2   cup shredded part-skim mozzarella cheese
- 1/2   cup light raspberry vinaigrette salad dressing

Toss together the spinach, strawberries, oranges, tomatoes, and cheese in a salad bowl. Add dressing and toss until thoroughly coated. Serve immediately.

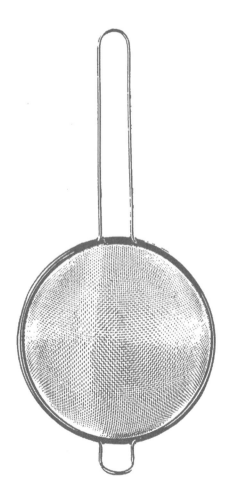

Exchanges
1 Fruit
1 Vegetable
1 1/2 Fat

Calories 158
   Calories from Fat........... 62
Total Fat 7   g
   Saturated Fat............... 1.6   g
   Trans Fat 0   g
Cholesterol 11   mg
Sodium 418   mg
Total Carbohydrate 19   g
   Dietary Fiber 4   g
   Sugars 13   g
Protein 7   g

Soul Food
Desserts

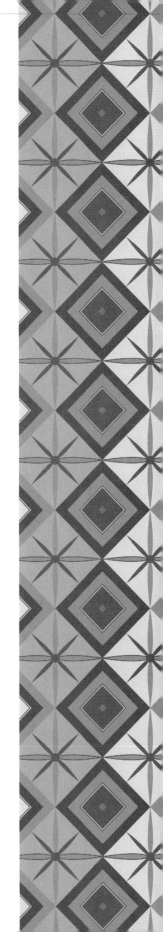

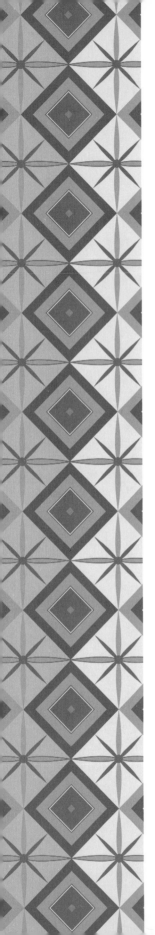

Althea's Frozen Fruit Cups

Preparation time: 20 min ✦ Serves 24 ✦ Serving size: 1 small fruit cup

8	oz fat-free cream cheese
1/2	cup sugar
1	10-oz jar maraschino cherries, drained
1	11-oz can mandarin oranges, drained
1	8-oz can crushed pineapple, drained
1/2	cup chopped pecans
8	oz lite whipped topping

1 In a mixing bowl, beat the cream cheese and sugar; mix until fluffy. Take 12 cherries and cut in half. Take remaining cherries and chop into small pieces. Take 24 orange segments and set aside.

2 Add pineapple, pecans, and chopped cherries to cream cheese mixture. Fold in whipped topping and remaining oranges. Line extra small muffin tin with muffin liners or foil liners.

3 Spoon fruit mixture into cups. Garnish with reserved cherries and oranges. Freeze until firm. Remove from freezer 10 minutes before serving.

Exchanges
1 Carbohydrate
1/2 Fat

Calories	82	
Calories from Fat	25	
Total Fat	3	g
Saturated Fat	1.2	g
Trans Fat	0	g
Cholesterol	1	mg
Sodium	67	mg
Total Carbohydrate	12	g
Dietary Fiber	1	g
Sugars	9	g
Protein	2	g

Angel Food Cake

Preparation time: 30 min ✦ Serves 14 ✦ Serving size: 1/14 slice

Cake

1	cup cake flour
3/4	cup Splenda® No Calorie Sweetener
1 1/4	cup egg whites (about 10 large egg whites) at room temperature
1 1/4	tsp cream of tartar
1/4	tsp salt
1	tsp vanilla extract

Sauce

3/4	cup mixed berries, such as raspberries and strawberries, fresh or frozen
1	Tbsp fresh lemon juice
3	Tbsp Splenda® No Calorie Sweetener or all-fruit jelly (not included in nutritional analysis)

1 Preheat the oven to 350°F. Sift the flour twice with 1/2 cup of the Splenda®. With an electric mixer on high speed, beat the egg whites, cream of tartar, and salt until soft peaks form when the mixer is removed from the batter. Add half of the remaining Splenda® sugar and beat for 1 minute. Add the remaining Splenda®, 2 Tbsp at a time, beating after each addition. Stir in the vanilla.

2 Fold the flour and Splenda® mixture into the egg whites, 1/4 cup at a time, until just incorporated. Put the batter in an ungreased 10-inch tube pan and bake at 350°F until the cake is light golden brown and springy to the touch, about 1 hour. Invert the pan and let the cake cool completely before removing from the pan.

3 Meanwhile, prepare the dessert sauce. Puree the berries in a blender with the lemon juice. Blend in the Splenda® by the tablespoonful, tasting after each addition. Strain through a fine strainer, pressing with a rubber spatula to release the juices. Place a slice of angel food cake on each plate. (Store the leftover cake in an airtight container or freeze for longer storage.) Drizzle the mixed berry sauce over the cake.

Exchanges
1 1/2 Carbohydrate

Calories	93
Calories from Fat	1
Total Fat	0 g
Saturated Fat	0 g
Trans Fat	0 g
Cholesterol	0 mg
Sodium	78 mg
Total Carbohydrate	19 g
Dietary Fiber	1 g
Sugars	11 g
Protein	3 g

Apple-Cranberry Pie

Preparation time: 30 min ✦ Serves 12 ✦ Serving size: 1 slice

1/4	cup brandy or apple juice
1	cup dried cranberries
2/3	cup Splenda® Sugar Blend for Baking
3	Tbsp all-purpose flour
1/4	tsp ground allspice
2 1/4	lb Granny Smith apples, peeled and thinly sliced
1	tsp vanilla extract
	Low-fat pie crust (see page 197)
	Reduced-sugar vanilla ice cream (optional)

Microwave the brandy or apple juice in a microwave-safe bowl at high power for 30 seconds; stir in dried cranberries. Cover mixture and let stand 10 minutes. Combine Splenda®, flour, and allspice in a large bowl; stir in cranberry mixture, apple slices, and vanilla. Prepare the low-fat pie crust by following directions on page 197. Press pastry into a pie pan and flute edges. Spoon apple-cranberry mixture into pie crust. Bake at 375°F for 1 hour, shielding edges of crust with aluminum foil after 30 minutes to prevent excessive browning. Cool pie on a wire rack 1 hour. Serve with a small scoop of reduced-sugar vanilla ice cream, if desired.

Exchanges
2 1/2 Carbohydrate

Calories	193	
Calories from Fat	27	
Total Fat	3	g
Saturated Fat	0.7	g
Trans Fat	0.3	g
Cholesterol	2	mg
Sodium	152	mg
Total Carbohydrate	39	g
Dietary Fiber	2	g
Sugars	28	g
Protein	2	g

Bread Pudding

Preparation time: 25 min ✦ Serves 16 ✦ Serving size: 2 × 2-inch square
with 1 Tbsp sauce

Pudding
2 Tbsp brandy
1/2 cup raisins
1 1/2 cup low-fat (1%) milk
1/2 cup Splenda® Sugar Blend for Baking
1 tsp vanilla flavoring
1 tsp walnut flavoring
1/4 tsp nutmeg
1/2 tsp cinnamon
1/16 tsp salt
3/4 cup egg substitute
6 1/2 oz French bread or day-old bread, broken into pieces

Sauce
1/2 cup Splenda® Sugar Blend for Baking
1/4 cup Karo syrup
1/4 cup light, soft, tub margarine
1/4 cup brandy

1 Combine brandy and raisins. Let sit for 30 minutes, until raisins become plump. Drain and reserve brandy.

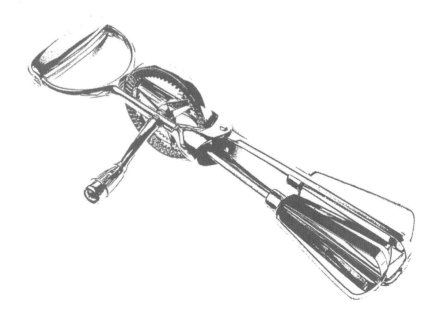

2 Take reserved liquid and mix with milk, Splenda®, vanilla and walnut flavorings, nutmeg, cinnamon, salt, and egg substitute. Mix well. Add broken bread pieces. Mix well; consistency should be similar to oatmeal. Pour into an 8-inch square baking dish. Sprinkle with the raisins. Chill ingredients for 30 minutes. Place baking dish in a water bath in a larger pan and cover. Bake at 350°F for 20 minutes; then uncover and bake for 10 more minutes.

3 Meanwhile, prepare the sauce. Combine the Splenda®, Karo syrup, and margarine and bring to a simmer over medium heat. When all ingredients have dissolved and combined, remove from heat and add brandy.

4 When a knife inserted into the center of the pudding comes out clean, remove from oven. Serve bread pudding with 1 Tbsp sauce.

Exchanges
2 Carbohydrate
1/2 Fat

Calories........................157
    Calories from Fat.......... 32
Total Fat .... 4 g
    Saturated Fat.............. 0.7 g
    Trans Fat .... 0.5 g
Cholesterol .... 1 mg
Sodium.........................134 mg
Total Carbohydrate ..... 27 g
    Dietary Fiber .... 0 g
    Sugars .... 21 g
Protein .... 3 g

Cool 'N' Easy Fruit Pie

Preparation time: 20 min ✦ Serves 8 ✦ Serving size: 1 slice

1	9-inch graham cracker crumb pie crust, baked
2/3	cup boiling water
1	0.3-oz pkg sugar-free gelatin dessert, any flavor
1/2	cup cold water
	Ice cubes
3 1/2	cups fat-free whipped topping
1	cup fresh raspberries

Bake the graham cracker crumb pie crust according to package instructions. In a large bowl, stir boiling water into gelatin mix, about 2 minutes or until dissolved. Mix cold water and enough ice cubes to make 1 1/4 cup. Add to gelatin; stir until slightly thickened. Remove any ice that has not melted. Gently stir in whipped topping using a wire whisk. Fold in raspberries. Refrigerate until mixture is very thick and will mound. Spoon into the baked pie crust. Refrigerate for 2 hours. Garnish with additional fruit.

Exchanges
2 Carbohydrate
1/2 Fat

Calories 174
    Calories from Fat 46
Total Fat .... 5 g
    Saturated Fat .... 1 g
    Trans Fat .... 0 g
Cholesterol .... 0 mg
Sodium .... 181 mg
Total Carbohydrate ..... 26 g
    Dietary Fiber .... 2 g
    Sugars .... 10 g
Protein .... 2 g

Cranberry Coffee Cake

Preparation time: 20 min ✦ Serves 12 ✦ Serving size: 1 slice

6	Tbsp light, soft, tub margarine
1/2	cup brown sugar
1 1/2	cups whole fresh cranberries
1/2	cup sugar
1	egg white
1 1/2	cups flour
2	tsp baking powder
1/2	cup low-fat (1%) milk

Mix 3 Tbsp margarine and brown sugar and press in bottom of an
8 × 8 × 2-inch pan. Pour the cranberries over this. Cream 3 Tbsp margarine
and sugar. Add egg white. Sift the flour and baking powder and add,
alternating with milk. Pour this mixture over the cranberries. Bake for
25 minutes at 400°F.

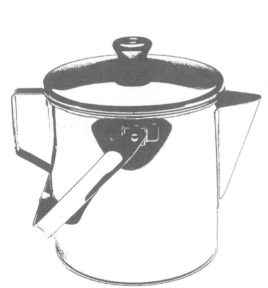

Exchanges
2 Carbohydrate

Calories........................ 156
   Calories from Fat........... 23
Total Fat .... 3 g
   Saturated Fat............... 0.3 g
   Trans Fat .... 0 g
Cholesterol .... 1 mg
Sodium..........................119 mg
Total Carbohydrate ......31 g
   Dietary Fiber .... 1 g
   Sugars .... 19 g
Protein .... 2 g

Fruit and Pasta

Preparation time: 20 min ✦ Serves 25 ✦ Serving size: 1/25 recipe

3/4	cup white sugar
3/4	cup egg substitute
2	Tbsp all-purpose flour
2	cups pineapple juice
1	Tbsp lemon juice
1	16-oz pkg acini di pepe pasta (like orzo)
2	20-oz cans pineapple chunks, drained
2	11-oz cans mandarin oranges, drained
3/4	cup maraschino cherries, chopped
1/2	lb miniature marshmallows
12	oz fat-free whipped topping, thawed

In large saucepan over low heat, combine the sugar, egg substitute, flour, pineapple juice, and lemon juice. Stir and cook until thickened. Remove from heat. While sauce is cooking, bring a large pot of water to a boil. Add pasta and cook for 8–10 minutes or until al dente; drain and rinse with cold water. In a large bowl, combine the cooked mixture with the pasta; toss to coat thoroughly. Refrigerate 8 hours or overnight. Toss pasta mix with the pineapple chunks, mandarin oranges, maraschino cherries, marshmallows, and whipped topping. Refrigerate until time to serve.

Exchanges
3 Carbohydrate

Calories	193	
Calories from Fat	3	
Total Fat	0	g
Saturated Fat	0	g
Trans Fat	0	g
Cholesterol	0	mg
Sodium	27	mg
Total Carbohydrate	43	g
Dietary Fiber	2	g
Sugars	27	g
Protein	3	g

Guava Cheesecake

Preparation time: 20 min ✦ Serves 12 ✦ Serving size: 1 slice

2	8-oz pkg fat-free cream cheese
1/2	cup sugar
1	tsp vanilla extract
1/2	cup egg substitute
1	9-inch graham cracker pie crust
4	Tbsp guava paste, melted, or guava jelly

In a mixing bowl, beat the cream cheese, sugar, and vanilla until smooth. Add egg substitute; beat on low speed. Pour into pie crust. Stir in guava paste or jam. Swirl until evenly distributed. Bake at 350°F for 30 minutes or until center is set. Cool for 1 hour. Refrigerate overnight. Let stand for 30 minutes before slicing.

Exchanges
2 Carbohydrate
1/2 Fat

Calories	187	
Calories from Fat	30	
Total Fat	3	g
Saturated Fat	0.7	g
Trans Fat	0	g
Cholesterol	7	mg
Sodium	496	mg
Total Carbohydrate	26	g
Dietary Fiber	1	g
Sugars	18	g
Protein	9	g

Heaven-Sent Cake

Preparation time: 20 min ✦ Serves 24 ✦ Serving size: 1 slice

Nonstick cooking spray
1 1/2 cups flour divided
2 tsp baking powder
1 tsp ground cinnamon
1/2 tsp ground nutmeg
1/2 tsp salt
1/4 tsp ground ginger
1 cup Splenda® Sugar Blend for Baking
9 Tbsp corn-oil stick margarine
2 Tbsp honey
6 eggs, separated
1/2 cup low-fat (1%) milk
1/2 cup slivered almonds
1 cup chopped dates
1 cup raisins
2 Tbsp flour

Preheat oven to 300°F. Spray a cake tube pan with nonstick cooking spray. Mix the flour, baking powder, cinnamon, nutmeg, salt, and ginger in a medium bowl. In another bowl, mix the Splenda®, margarine, and honey; beat until fluffy. Add egg yolks one at a time, beating well after each addition. Add flour mixture alternately with milk. Beat until smooth. Beat egg whites in another large bowl until peaks are formed. Stir egg whites into the batter. Toss in almonds, dates, raisins, and the 2 Tbsp of flour. Pour into the prepared pan. Bake 2 hours and 45 minutes. Cool 10 minutes. Loosen from sides of pan and remove cake. Cool before serving. Slice very thin.

Exchanges
2 Carbohydrate
1 Fat

Calories..........................182
    Calories from Fat........... 64
Total Fat .... 7 g
    Saturated Fat................ 1.4 g
    Trans Fat .... 0.8 g
Cholesterol .... 53 mg
Sodium..........................144 mg
Total Carbohydrate ..... 27 g
    Dietary Fiber .... 1 g
    Sugars .... 19 g
Protein .... 4 g

Hebni Banana Pudding

Preparation time: 20 min ✦ Serves 30 ✦ Serving size: 1/30 recipe

 2 1-oz pkg sugar-free, fat-free vanilla pudding mix
 4 cups low-fat (1%) milk
16 oz fat-free whipped topping
 8 medium bananas, cut into pieces
 1 cup orange juice
 2 12-oz boxes reduced-fat vanilla wafers

Prepare the vanilla pudding according to package instructions, using the low-fat milk; set aside and chill for 5 minutes. Add softened whipped topping and mix well. In a separate bowl, add the bananas and orange juice. Drain the orange juice from the bananas and discard the juice. In a trifle bowl, layer the vanilla wafers, bananas, and pudding until you reach the top. The pudding goes on last, and garnish by crumbling remaining vanilla wafers over the top of the pudding. Chill and serve in shot glasses or in small martini glasses.

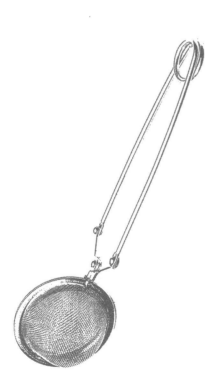

Exchanges
2 Carbohydrate
1/2 Fat

Calories.........................175
   Calories from Fat........... 28
Total Fat .... 3 g
   Saturated Fat............... 1.4 g
   Trans Fat .... 0 g
Cholesterol .... 2 mg
Sodium.........................148 mg
Total Carbohydrate ..... 34 g
   Dietary Fiber .... 1 g
   Sugars ....18 g
Protein .... 2 g

Lemon Angel Trifle

Preparation time: 10 min ✦ Serves 10 ✦ Serving size: 1/10 recipe

> 1 0.3-oz pkg sugar-free lemon gelatin
> 8 oz lite whipped topping
> 1 prepared angel food cake (about 12 oz)
>   *Garnish*: 5 medium strawberries

Sprinkle the gelatin over whipped topping; mix and set aside. Break angel food cake into small walnut-size pieces. In a serving bowl, layer the angel food cake and lemon whipped topping, ending with whipped topping. Garnish with strawberries.

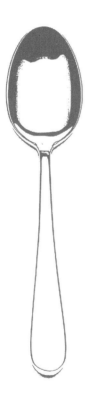

Exchanges
2 Carbohydrate

Calories.........................130
   Calories from Fat............. 3
Total Fat .... 0 g
   Saturated Fat.................. 0 g
   Trans Fat .... 0 g
Cholesterol .... 0 mg
Sodium......................... 290 mg
Total Carbohydrate ..... 28 g
   Dietary Fiber .... 1 g
   Sugars .... 3 g
Protein .... 3 g

Lemon Berry Crunch Parfaits

Preparation time: 15 min ✦ Serves 10 ✦ Serving size: 1/2 cup

8 oz lite whipped topping, thawed
3 6-oz containers fat-free, sugar-free lemon yogurt
2 cups blueberries
2 cups low-fat granola cereal

In a large bowl, fold the whipped topping into the yogurt with a wire whisk until smooth. Alternating, layer the whipped topping mixture, blueberries, and cereal in 10 (6-oz) dessert glasses. Refrigerate until ready to serve.

Exchanges
2 Carbohydrate

Calories 141
  Calories from Fat 9
Total Fat .... 1 g
  Saturated Fat .... 0.3 g
  Trans Fat .... 0 g
Cholesterol .... 1 mg
Sodium .... 83 mg
Total Carbohydrate ..... 29 g
  Dietary Fiber .... 2 g
  Sugars .... 12 g
Protein .... 3 g

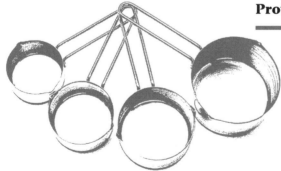

Lemon Rice Cake

Preparation time: 20 min ✦ Serves 16 ✦ Serving size: 1 slice

4	cups nonfat milk
1 3/4	cups short-grain rice
	tsp vanilla extract
1/4	cup raisins
1/4	cup rum or rum extract
	Nonstick cooking spray
2–3	Tbsp cornmeal, for dusting
3/4	cup sugar
	Grated rind of 1 large lemon
3	Tbsp corn oil margarine, diced
3	eggs
2–3	Tbsp lemon juice (*optional*)
2	Tbsp rum
1/2	cup lite whipped topping

1 Bring the milk to a boil. Sprinkle in the rice and bring back to a boil. Add the vanilla extract, lower the heat, and simmer, stirring occasionally, for 30 minutes.

2 Meanwhile, bring the raisins and rum to a boil; then set aside.

3 Spray the bottom and sides of a 10-inch loose-bottomed cake pan with nonstick cooking spray. Dust with the cornmeal and shake out any excess.

4 Remove the rice from the heat and stir in all but 1 Tbsp of sugar, the lemon rind, and the margarine. Stir until the sugar is dissolved. Place in water to cool. Stir in the soaked raisins and rum.

5 Beat the eggs with an electric mixer for about 2 minutes, until light and foamy. Gradually beat in about half the rice mixture, then stir in the rest. Stir in lemon juice, if desired. Pour mixture into the prepared pan and smooth the top. Sprinkle with the reserved 1 Tbsp sugar and bake in a preheated oven at 325°F for about 40 minutes, until risen and golden. Cool in the pan on a wire rack.

6 Make the topping. Mix 2 Tbsp rum into 1/2 cup lite whipped topping, and serve on cake slices.

Exchanges
2 Carbohydrate
1 Fat

Calories..........................191
   Calories from Fat...........31
Total Fat .... 3 g
   Saturated Fat.................. 1 g
   Trans Fat .... 0.4 g
Cholesterol .... 41 mg
Sodium.......................... 63 mg
Total Carbohydrate ..... 33 g
   Dietary Fiber .... 1 g
   Sugars ....14 g
Protein .... 5 g

Lemon Squares

Preparation time: 15 min ✦ Serves 75 ✦ Serving size: 2 × 1-inch rectangle

Crust

1/2 lb corn-oil margarine, softened (about 2 sticks)
2 tsp butter extract
1/2 cup confectioners' sugar
2 cups unbleached flour
Pinch of salt

Topping

1 cup egg substitute
1/2 cups granulated sugar
2 tsp butter flavoring
6 Tbsp unbleached flour
6 Tbsp freshly squeezed lemon juice
6 Tbsp finely grated lemon zest
Confectioners' sugar for topping

1 Adjust the oven rack to the middle shelf. Preheat the oven to 350°F. Prepare the crust. Combine the margarine, butter extract, confectioners' sugar, flour, and salt; blend with your fingers or a pastry blender. Pat evenly into a 10 × 15-inch jelly roll pan. Bake for 15–18 minutes until firm.

2 Meanwhile, beat the egg substitute slightly; stir in the sugar, butter flavoring, flour, lemon juice, and lemon zest. Mix well and spread over the baked crust. Bake for 20–25 minutes more, until the topping is firm.

3 Let stand until cool. Cut into 2 × 1-inch rectangles, or 1 1/4-inch squares for petit fours. The lemon squares can be refrigerated or frozen, tightly wrapped, at that point. To serve, let the cookies defrost in the refrigerator if frozen. Sprinkle the top with confectioners' sugar.

Exchanges
1/2 Carbohydrate
1/2 Fat

Calories............................ 57
   Calories from Fat........... 22
Total Fat .... 2 g
   Saturated Fat................ 0.5 g
   Trans Fat .... 0.4 g
Cholesterol .... 0 mg
Sodium.......................... 43 mg
Total Carbohydrate .... 8 g
   Dietary Fiber .... 0 g
   Sugars .... 5 g
Protein .... 1 g

Lite Brownies

Preparation time: 30 min ✦ Serves 16 ✦ Serving size: 2 × 2-inch square

- 6 Tbsp unsweetened cocoa
- 1 cup Splenda® Sugar Blend for Baking
- 1/2 cup corn-oil stick margarine
- 1/2 cup egg substitute
- 1/2 cup self-rising flour
- 1 Tbsp vanilla extract
- 1/2 cup chopped toasted pecans
  Garnish: powdered sugar

Combine cocoa and Splenda®. Add margarine, egg substitute, flour, vanilla, and pecans, stirring until just combined. Pour mixture into a lightly greased 8-inch square pan. Bake at 350°F for 25–30 minutes. Cool. Cut into 2-inch squares, and dust with powdered sugar before serving.

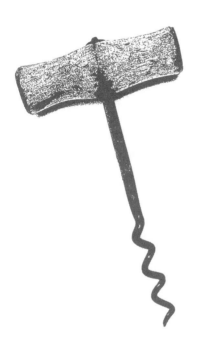

Exchanges
1 Carbohydrate
1 1/2 Fat

Calories..........................148
   Calories from Fat........... 77
Total Fat .... 9 g
   Saturated Fat............... 1.4 g
   Trans Fat .... 1.0 g
Cholesterol .... 0 mg
Sodium......................... 123 mg
Total Carbohydrate ......17 g
   Dietary Fiber .... 1 g
   Sugars .... 12 g
Protein .... 2 g

Low-Fat Pie Crust

Preparation time: 15 min ✦ Serves 10 ✦ Serving size: 1 slice

2   Tbsp corn-oil stick margarine
2   Tbsp reduced-fat cream cheese
2   Tbsp Splenda® No Calorie Sweetener
1   tsp vanilla extract
1   Tbsp low-fat (1%) milk
1/4 cup egg substitute
1   cup flour
1/2 tsp baking powder
1/2 tsp salt

1 Combine first 4 ingredients and beat at medium speed until smooth. Add the milk and egg substitute. In a separate bowl, combine flour, baking powder, and salt. Mix well. Add dry ingredients to wet ingredients.

2 Press together and mix well. Wrap dough with plastic wrap. Chill for 15 minutes. While dough is still in plastic wrap, roll out into a circle. If the dough is too soft, add a little flour; if the dough is too dry, add a little more milk. Freeze it for 5 minutes to help remove the plastic wrap. Remove dough from freezer and place in a pie pan. Press dough into bottom and sides of pan.

Exchanges
1/2 Starch
1 Fat

Calories 79
  Calories from Fat 27
Total Fat .... 3 g
  Saturated Fat .... 0.9 g
  Trans Fat .... 0.4 g
Cholesterol .... 2 mg
Sodium ....182 mg
Total Carbohydrate ..... 10 g
  Dietary Fiber .... 0 g
  Sugars .... 1 g
Protein .... 2 g

Mango Cheesecake

Preparation time: 20 min ✦ Serves 10 ✦ Serving size: 1 slice

> 15 oz low-fat ricotta cheese
> 1 1/2 lb fat-free cream cheese, soft
> 1 cup Splenda® Sugar Blend for Baking
> 1/4 cup flour
> 1 1/2 tsp almond flavoring
> 1/4 tsp salt
> 3 egg whites
> 2 cups pureed mango
> *Garnish:* chopped mango

1 Preheat oven to 400°F. Puree the ricotta cheese in a blender on medium speed until smooth. Add cream cheese to blender. Transfer to a mixing bowl.

2 Add Splenda®, flour, almond extract, and salt. Mix well. Add egg whites; mix on low speed until it is mixed well. Remove 1/3 cup batter and set aside. On low speed, add mango to the remaining batter.

3 Pour the batter into a spring-form pan. Take the reserved batter and put four large spoonfuls of batter on top of fruit batter. Swirl the white batter with the fruit batter softly. Do not overwork the batter.

4 Bake for 1 hour at 400°F. Let cool down in warm oven to prevent cracking. Refrigerate for 4 hours. Serve chilled. Garnish with chopped mango.

Exchanges
2 1/2 Carbohydrate
1 Lean Meat

Calories........................ 236
  Calories from Fat........... 20
Total Fat .... 2 g
  Saturated Fat............... 1.4 g
  Trans Fat .... 0 g
Cholesterol .... 22 mg
Sodium......................... 642 mg
Total Carbohydrate ..... 36 g
  Dietary Fiber .... 1 g
  Sugars .... 30 g
Protein ....16 g

Mango Cream

Preparation time: 10 min ✦ Serves 15 ✦ Serving size: 1/3 cup

- 3 lb ripe mangoes
- 4–5 Tbsp lime juice, depending on sweetness of mangoes
- 1 cup lite whipped topping

1 Peel the mangoes; remove the flesh from the pits and puree in a food processor. Stir in the lime juice.

2 Fold the whipped topping into the mango puree until the mixture is smooth. Spoon mixture into small wine glasses. Refrigerate for several hours or overnight. Serve cold.

Exchanges
1 Fruit

Calories 52
   Calories from Fat 6
Total Fat .... 1 g
   Saturated Fat .... 0.6 g
   Trans Fat .... 0 g
Cholesterol .... 0 mg
Sodium .... 3 mg
Total Carbohydrate ..... 12 g
   Dietary Fiber .... 1 g
   Sugars .... 10 g
Protein .... 0 g

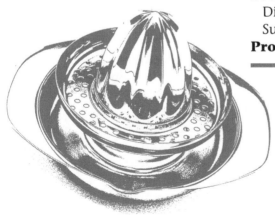

Mango Upside-Down Cake

Preparation time: 20 min ✦ Serves 12 ✦ Serving size: 1 slice

   Nonstick cooking spray
2 slightly underripe mangoes, peeled and sliced
2/3 cup sugar
   Juice and rind of 1 lemon or lime
1 egg
5 Tbsp light, soft, tub margarine
1 cup flour
3/4 cup sugar
1 tsp baking powder
1/4 tsp salt
2 egg yolks, well beaten
1/4 cup milk
2 egg whites, beaten stiff

1 Coat an 8-inch pie pan or ovenproof dish with nonstick cooking spray. Cover with peeled and thick-sliced mangoes. Sprinkle with 2/3 cup sugar and lemon or lime juice and rind. Beat an egg, pour over fruit, and dot with 4 Tbsp margarine.

2 Sift the flour with 1/2 cup sugar, baking powder, and salt. Add well-beaten egg yolks, 1 Tbsp melted margarine, and 1/4 cup milk. Beat well and cover fruit with this batter.

3 Bake in a preheated oven at 425°F for 30 minutes. Reverse it on an ovenproof platter and cool slightly. Beat 2 egg whites until stiff and add slowly to 1/4 cup sugar. Cover the cake with this meringue and bake slowly at 300°F for 15 minutes or until brown. Serve warm.

Exchanges
2 1/2 Carbohydrate

Calories 188
   Calories from Fat........... 27
Total Fat .... 3 g
   Saturated Fat............... 0.7 g
   Trans Fat .... 0 g
Cholesterol .... 53 mg
Sodium .... 129 mg
Total Carbohydrate ..... 38 g
   Dietary Fiber .... 1 g
   Sugars .... 29 g
Protein .... 3 g

New-Fashioned Vanilla Custard

Preparation time: 15 min ✦ Serves 6 ✦ Serving size: 2/3 cup

1	pkg instant sugar-free vanilla pudding or pie-filling mix
1 1/2	cups nonfat milk
1	cup fat-free sour cream
1	cup fresh strawberries, raspberries, blueberries, or blackberries

Place instant pudding mix in a medium bowl. With a wire whisk, stir in the milk until mixture is smooth and slightly thickened. Add sour cream and whisk until smooth. Cover. Refrigerate at least 1 hour. Spoon custard into six individual dessert dishes; top with assorted berries.

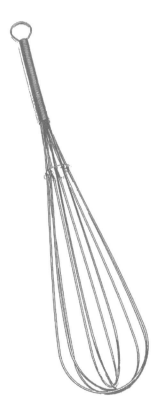

Exchanges
1 Carbohydrate

Calories 77
   Calories from Fat 1
Total Fat .... 0 g
   Saturated Fat .... 0 g
   Trans Fat .... 0 g
Cholesterol .... 5 mg
Sodium .... 252 mg
Total Carbohydrate ..... 10 g
   Dietary Fiber .... 1 g
   Sugars .... 6 g
Protein .... 5 g

Orange Cake

Preparation time: 20 min ✦ Serves 16 ✦ Serving size: 1 small slice

	Nonstick cooking spray
1/2	cup corn-oil stick margarine, softened
3/4	cup sugar
3	eggs, beaten
2	medium oranges, juiced and zested
1 1/4	cups self-rising flour
3	Tbsp ground almonds
3	Tbsp fat-free half and half

Glaze

6	Tbsp fresh-squeezed orange juice
2	Tbsp sugar

1 Grease a round 7-inch cake pan with nonstick cooking spray.

2 Cream the margarine and 3/4 cup sugar until fluffy. Add eggs one at a time, beating thoroughly after each addition. Add zest of two oranges. Gently fold in self-rising flour, ground almonds, and half and half.

3 Place batter in a cake pan and bake at 350°F for 55 minutes or until a skewer inserted in the center comes out clean.

4 Meanwhile, prepare the glaze. Place the orange juice and sugar into a pot and bring mixture to a boil. Simmer for 5 minutes.

5 Transfer the finished cake to a serving plate, and drizzle the glaze over it until completely absorbed.

Exchanges
1 1/2 Carbohydrate
1 Fat

Calories	160	
Calories from Fat	68	
Total Fat	8	g
Saturated Fat	1.4	g
Trans Fat	1	g
Cholesterol	40	mg
Sodium	198	mg
Total Carbohydrate	21	g
Dietary Fiber	0	g
Sugars	13	g
Protein	3	g

Peach Pear Fruit Compote

Preparation time: 10 min ✦ Serves 6 ✦ Serving size: 1 cup

- 1/2 cup water
- 1 1-lb bag fresh cranberries
- 1/2 cup Splenda® No Calorie Sweetener
- 1 15-oz can sliced peaches, packed in extra-light syrup
- 1 15-oz can pears, packed in extra-light syrup
- 2 Tbsp fresh lemon juice
- 1/4 tsp ground cinnamon
- 1/4 tsp ground nutmeg
  Garnish: orange rind strips

Heat 1/2 cup water in a large pot, add cranberries, and bring to a boil. The cranberries will burst with heat. Pour the Splenda® over cranberries; continue to heat until it dissolves. Add the peaches and pears with syrup, lemon juice, cinnamon, and nutmeg, stirring constantly over high heat. Remove from heat. Serve in decorative bowl or individual containers. Garnish with orange rind strips, if desired.

Exchanges
2 Fruit

Calories	112	
Calories from Fat	2	
Total Fat	0	g
Saturated Fat	0	g
Trans Fat	0	g
Cholesterol	0	mg
Sodium	8	mg
Total Carbohydrate	29	g
Dietary Fiber	5	g
Sugars	22	g
Protein	1	g

Rojean's Award-Winning Cheesecake Parfait

Preparation time: 10 min ✦ Serves 24 ✦ Serving size: 1 parfait glass

1	8-oz pkg reduced-fat cream cheese
1	8-oz pkg fat-free cream cheese
1	12-oz container fat-free whipped topping
2	Tbsp lemon juice
1	Tbsp vanilla flavoring
1/2	cup Splenda® Sugar Blend for Baking
1	24-oz can sugar-free pie filling, blueberry or cherry
	Garnish: mint leaves

Using a mixer, blend the cream cheese until whipped smooth; then add whipped topping, lemon juice, and vanilla flavoring. Layer 2 Tbsp cream cheese mixture in a parfait glass, and then add 2 Tbsp pie filling on top. Garnish with pie filling and mint leaves.

Exchanges
1 Carbohydrate
1/2 Fat

Calories............................ 95
    Calories from Fat............18
Total Fat .... 2 g
    Saturated Fat................ 1.3 g
    Trans Fat .... 0 g
Cholesterol .... 9 mg
Sodium..........................181 mg
Total Carbohydrate .... 13 g
    Dietary Fiber .... 1 g
    Sugars .... 8 g
Protein .... 4 g

Shorty's Blackberry Dumplings

Preparation time: 15 min ✦ Serves 6 ✦ Serving size: 1/2 cup fruit + 2 dumplings

1	quart frozen blackberries, no sugar added
1	cup + 2 tsp Splenda® No Calorie Sweetener
1/2	tsp lemon extract
3/4	tsp salt, divided
1	cup all-purpose flour
1	tsp baking powder
1/4	tsp ground nutmeg
2/3	cup low-fat (1%) milk
	Lite whipped topping (*optional*)

Bring the blackberries, 1 cup Splenda®, lemon extract, and 1/4 tsp salt to a boil on stovetop. Reduce heat and simmer 5 minutes. Do not overcook the berries. In a bowl, combine the remaining 1/2 tsp salt, flour, baking powder, 2 tsp Splenda®, and nutmeg in a medium bowl; stir in milk until just blended (dough will be thick). Drop dough by tablespoonfuls onto the hot blackberry mixture. Steam in a large stovetop pot until dumplings have doubled in size. Serve with a small dollop of whipped topping, if desired.

Exchanges
2 1/2 Carbohydrate

Calories	169	
Calories from Fat	9	
Total Fat	1	g
Saturated Fat	0.2	g
Trans Fat	0	g
Cholesterol	1	mg
Sodium	366	mg
Total Carbohydrate	37	g
Dietary Fiber	6	g
Sugars	14	g
Protein	4	g

Sistah's Peach Cobbler

Preparation time: 30 min ✦ Serves 14 ✦ Serving size: 1/14 recipe

Filling
- 2 large (29-oz) cans peaches, packed in light syrup, sliced, and drained
- 1/4 cup Splenda® Brown Sugar Blend
- 7 Tbsp tapioca
- 1 1/4 tsp cinnamon
- 1 tsp lemon juice
- 1 tsp vanilla

Crust
- 1 cup flour
- 1/2 cup Splenda® Sugar Blend for Baking
- 1 tsp baking powder
- 1/3 tsp salt
- 1/2 cup corn-oil stick margarine
- 1/2 cup egg substitute

Caramel sauce
- 1/4 cup Splenda® Brown Sugar Blend
- 2 Tbsp flour
- 1/8 tsp salt
- 1/4 cup light, soft, tub margarine
- 2 Tbsp lemon juice

1 Prepare the filling. Drain peaches, reserving 1/2 cup syrup for the sauce. In a large bowl, combine the peaches, Splenda® brown sugar, tapioca, cinnamon, lemon juice, and vanilla. Mix well and pour into an oblong baking dish.

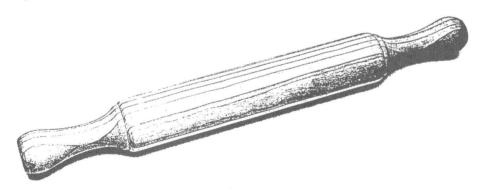

2 Prepare the crust. In a separate bowl, combine the flour, Splenda®, baking powder, and salt. Add margarine and mix until it resembles crumbs. Stir in egg substitute. Drop by spoonfuls on top of the peaches. Spread evenly. Bake at 350°F for 50 minutes. Cool.

3 Meanwhile, prepare the sauce. In a small saucepan, combine the Splenda® brown sugar, flour, salt, margarine, and reserved peach syrup. Bring to a boil over medium heat; stir for 1 minute or until thick. Remove from heat and add lemon juice.

4 Spoon the warm sauce over each individual serving of warm cobbler. Serve.

Exchanges
2 1/2 Carbohydrate
1/2 Fat

Calories 194
    Calories from Fat........... 42
Total Fat .... 5 g
    Saturated Fat............... 0.7 g
    Trans Fat .... 0.6 g
Cholesterol .... 0 mg
Sodium ....181 mg
Total Carbohydrate ..... 34 g
    Dietary Fiber .... 1 g
    Sugars .... 21 g
Protein .... 2 g

Snacking Cake

Preparation time: 20 min ✦ Serves 12 ✦ Serving size: 1 slice

1/2	cup corn-oil stick margarine
1/2	cup granulated sugar
1	tsp cinnamon
3/4	cup egg substitute
4	Tbsp rum
1 1/4	cups all-purpose flour
	Pinch salt

1 Preheat oven to 350°F. Lightly grease 10-inch spring-form cake pan. Place margarine, sugar, and cinnamon in a bowl; cream together. Add 1/4 cup egg substitute and beat well with an electric beater. Add remaining egg substitute, 1/4 cup at a time, beating well after each addition. Add rum. Mix flour with salt; stir into batter and mix with spatula until smooth.

2 Pour batter into the prepared cake pan and bake for 40–45 minutes, or until a toothpick inserted into the center comes out clean. Cool in the pan for about 10–15 minutes before transferring the cake to a wire rack for continued cooling. Garnish with powdered (confectioner's) sugar or with one of your favorite fruits.

Exchanges
1 Carbohydrate
1 1/2 Fat

Calories	158	
Calories from Fat	70	
Total Fat	8	g
Saturated Fat	1.4	g
Trans Fat	1.4	g
Cholesterol	0	mg
Sodium	118	mg
Total Carbohydrate	19	g
Dietary Fiber	0	g
Sugars	9	g
Protein	3	g

Strawberry Lime Dessert

Preparation time: 20 min ✦ Serves 6 ✦ Serving size: 3/4 cup

2	cups boiling water, divided
1	pkg sugar-free lime-flavored gelatin dessert
1/2	cup cold water
1	6-oz container nonfat vanilla yogurt
1	pkg sugar-free strawberry-flavored gelatin dessert
1	10-oz pkg frozen strawberries, unsweetened

1 In a medium bowl, stir 1 cup of the boiling water into lime gelatin, stirring 2 minutes or until completely dissolved. Stir in cold water. Refrigerate about 45 minutes or until slightly thickened (consistency of unbeaten egg whites).

2 Stir in the yogurt with a wire whisk until smooth. Pour into 2-quart serving bowl. Refrigerate for about 15 minutes or until set but not firm (mixture should stick to a finger when touched).

3 In a medium bowl, stir remaining 1 cup boiling water into strawberry gelatin, stirring 2 minutes or until completely dissolved. Stir in frozen strawberries until separated and gelatin is thickened.

4 Spoon strawberry mixture over lime gelatin mixture. Refrigerate for 2 hours or until firm. Serve. Store leftover dessert in refrigerator.

Exchanges
1/2 Carbohydrate

Calories	37	
Calories from Fat	0	
Total Fat	0	g
Saturated Fat	0	g
Trans Fat	0	g
Cholesterol	1	mg
Sodium	90	mg
Total Carbohydrate	6	g
Dietary Fiber	1	g
Sugars	4	g
Protein	3	g

Strawberry Shortcakes

Preparation time: 30 min ✦ Serves 10 ✦ Serving size: 1 biscuit plus 1/2 cup berries, sauce, and topping

    1 cup lite whipped topping
       Nonstick cooking spray
    1 7.5-oz container lower-fat refrigerated breakfast biscuits
4 1/2 cups diced strawberries
    2 Tbsp Splenda® Sugar Blend for Baking

1 Preheat oven to 400°F. Coat a baking sheet with nonstick spray. Bake biscuits at 400°F for 10–13 minutes, until golden. Cool on rack.

2 Prepare the strawberry sauce. Puree 2 cups diced strawberries mixed with the Splenda®.

3 Spoon 2 Tbsp sauce onto each of 10 plates. Slice each biscuit in half horizontally. Place bottom half on dishes. Spoon 1/4 cup berries on each. Dollop with whipped topping; cover with biscuit top. Garnish with whipped topping and sauce.

Exchanges
1 1/2 Carbohydrate

Calories.........................103
   Calories from Fat...........16
Total Fat .... 2 g
   Saturated Fat............... 0.9 g
   Trans Fat .... 0 g
Cholesterol .... 0 mg
Sodium.........................192 mg
Total Carbohydrate ..... 20 g
   Dietary Fiber .... 2 g
   Sugars .... 9 g
Protein .... 2 g

Sugar-Free Sorbet

Preparation time: 30 min ✦ Serves 8 ✦ Serving size: 3/4 cup

3 cups water

1 cup Splenda® No Calorie Sweetener

5 cups fresh or frozen sliced strawberries
(other seasonal fruits can be substituted)

2 Tbsp lemon juice

Bring 3 cups water and Splenda® to a boil in a medium saucepan over high heat, stirring until Splenda® dissolves. Remove from heat. Cool. In a blender, process this sugar syrup and the strawberries, in batches, until smooth. Stir in lemon juice. Cover. Pour mixture into the freezer container of a 1-gallon ice-cream maker and freeze according to manufacturer's instructions.

Exchanges
1/2 Carbohydrate

Calories........................... 43
   Calories from Fat............. 4
Total Fat .... 0 g
   Saturated Fat.................. 0 g
   Trans Fat .... 0 g
Cholesterol .... 0 mg
Sodium............................. 4 mg
Total Carbohydrate ..... 10 g
   Dietary Fiber .... 2 g
   Sugars .... 8 g
Protein .... 1 g

Church Recipes
The New Kitchen Ministry

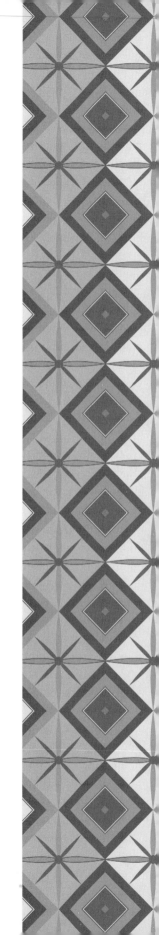

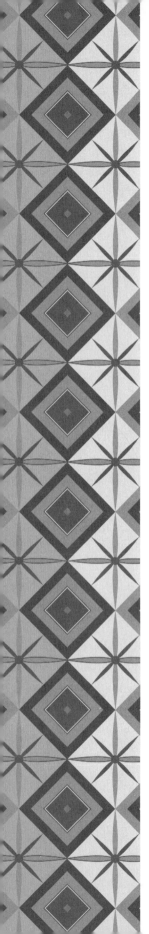

As part of its ongoing commitment to reduce health care disparities among Americans, the black church has become a vehicle for creating healthy lifestyle changes and promoting healthy eating habits among its members and communities. Nationwide, it has become popular for faith-based organizations to encourage African Americans to eat a healthy diet as part of an active lifestyle. Many of the recommendations that are encouraged include ideas such as "A Celebration of Healthy Eating and Living," promoting the national recommendation for Americans to eat 5–9 servings of fruits and vegetables a day for better health.

Many organizations have implemented programs that promote strategies endorsed and promoted by the pastor. The role of the pastor is crucial for church wellness because he or she can promote healthy living and lifestyle habits based on biblical principles. Ministries are used as a vehicle to promote health messages through the implementation of formal health ministries or committees. Health and kitchen ministries are fruitful environments for positive changes in the black community, and they are vital to the health of many African-American families.

To help do our part, we have provided several recipes to bring healthy eating and a healthy lifestyle to your church. Each recipe is designed to serve large groups in a healthful way. Next time you go to church, try bringing along at least one of these tasty, healthy recipes. These recipes do not have preparation times because the recipes are large enough that it may be best to have someone provide much-needed help in the kitchen. Depending on how many people you can get involved in this family activity, preparation times will vary.

Baked Scrambled Eggs

Serves 50 ✦ Serving size: 1/50 recipe

  45 egg whites
   5 egg yolks
   1 quart nonfat milk
   1 tsp salt
  14 oz fat-free cheddar cheese, shredded

Beat egg whites and yolks thoroughly. Add milk and salt. Mix until well blended. Pour egg mixture into a nonstick pan. Bake 20 minutes at 350°F. Remove from oven and sprinkle cheese over pan. Cheese will melt with heat from eggs. Serve hot.

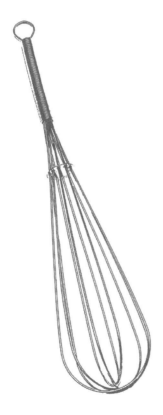

Exchanges
1 Very Lean Meat

Calories 40
    Calories from Fat 5
Total Fat .... 1 g
    Saturated Fat .... 0.2 g
    Trans Fat .... 0 g
Cholesterol .... 23 mg
Sodium .... 187 mg
Total Carbohydrate .... 2 g
    Dietary Fiber .... 0 g
    Sugars .... 2 g
Protein .... 7 g

Beef or Chicken Stock

Serves 80 ✦ Serving size: 1 cup

10 lb beef bones or chicken bones
10 gallons water
2 lb onions, chopped
1 lb celery, chopped
1 bunch parsley, chopped
Salt and pepper to taste

Simmer all ingredients on a stove until the vegetables have become tender and the bones have infused the stock with flavor. You can use this stock for beef or poultry gravies or any recipe that calls for a beef or chicken stock. This should be a low-sodium stock for all of your purposes.

Exchanges
Free Food

Calories........................... 12
  Calories from Fat............. 3
Total Fat .... 0 g
  Saturated Fat.................. 0 g
  Trans Fat .... 0 g
Cholesterol .... 4 mg
Sodium.......................... 64 mg
Total Carbohydrate .... 1 g
  Dietary Fiber .... 0 g
  Sugars .... 0 g
Protein .... 1 g

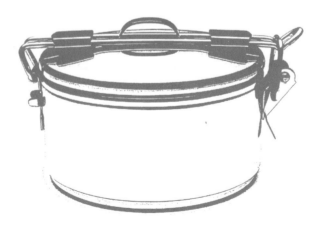

Carrot Cake

Serves 50 ✦ Serving size: 1 slice

2 3/4	lb	Splenda® Sugar Blend for Baking
1 3/4	lb	flour
2 1/2	Tbsp	baking soda
1	Tbsp + 1 tsp	salt
4	Tbsp + 1/3 tsp	cinnamon
1	Tbsp	baking powder
2 1/2	cups	canola oil
3	cups	egg substitute
3	lb	grated carrots

Mix dry ingredients together in a large mixing bowl. Add oil to dry mix and mix well. Mix until smooth. Add egg substitute. Add grated carrots and mix well at medium speed. Bake at 350°F. Makes six layers for three cakes. Serve this splendid cake with the cream cheese icing on page 219.

Exchanges
2 1/2 Carbohydrate
2 Fat

Calories	224	
Calories from Fat	52	
Total Fat	6	g
Saturated Fat	0.4	g
Trans Fat	0	g
Cholesterol	0	mg
Sodium	353	mg
Total Carbohydrate	39	g
Dietary Fiber	1	g
Sugars	26	g
Protein	3	g

Collard Greens
with Smoked Turkey

Serves 50 ✦ Serving size: 1/50 recipe

12	lb fresh collard greens
2	lb smoked turkey necks
4	cubes chicken bouillon
1	gallon water
3	whole onions, chopped
4	garlic cloves, chopped
	Splenda® No Calorie Sweetener to taste
	Hot pepper flakes *(optional)*

Take the stems off the greens and tear into small pieces. Wash very well, drain, and rinse again. Place all ingredients in a very large pot, cover with water, and cook until tender, about 4 hours. Add water as needed while cooking. Add a little Splenda® to taste to take the bitterness out of the greens and some hot pepper flakes as desired. Serve with necks.

Exchanges
1 Vegetable

Calories 27
   Calories from Fat 2
Total Fat .... 0 g
   Saturated Fat .... 0 g
   Trans Fat .... 0 g
Cholesterol .... 0 mg
Sodium .... 149 mg
Total Carbohydrate .... 6 g
   Dietary Fiber .... 2 g
   Sugars .... 1 g
Protein .... 1 g

Cream Cheese Icing

Serves 50 ✦ Serving size: 1/50 recipe

- 1 lb fat-free cream cheese
- 1/2 lb light, soft, tub margarine
- 2 Tbsp Splenda® No Calorie Sweetener
- 4 Tbsp + 1/3 tsp vanilla
- 1/4 cup low-fat milk (*optional*)

Cream the cream cheese and margarine. Add Splenda® until icing obtains the body needed for spreading. Add vanilla; blend for 1 minute until light and fluffy. Add low-fat milk to obtain the right consistency if needed.

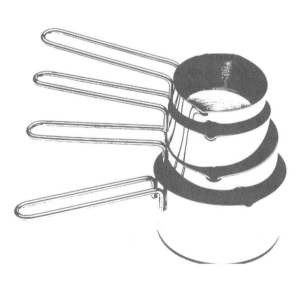

Exchanges
1/2 Fat

Calories......................... 24
   Calories from Fat.......... 13
Total Fat .... 1 g
   Saturated Fat.................0.1 g
   Trans Fat .... 0 g
Cholesterol .... 1 mg
Sodium.......................... 93 mg
Total Carbohydrate .... 1 g
   Dietary Fiber .... 0 g
   Sugars .... 0 g
Protein .... 1 g

Deacon Board's Chicken

Serves 40 ✦ Serving size: 1/40 recipe

Marinade

1 quart lite soy sauce
1 quart sherry wine
2 quarts pineapple juice
1 quart red wine vinegar
1/8 cup fresh garlic
1 lb Splenda® Sugar Blend for Baking
40 boneless skinless chicken parts

Sauce

1 cup light, soft, tub margarine
1 cup flour
2 quarts pineapple juice
1 quart sherry wine
1 quart red wine vinegar

1 Prepare the marinade. In a mixing bowl, blend together the soy sauce, sherry wine, pineapple juice, vinegar, garlic, and Splenda®. Pour marinade over boneless chicken parts and let stand in the refrigerator for 4–6 hours. Remove chicken parts from marinade and place on sheet pan. Discard marinade. Bake in an oven at 350ºF for 45 minutes, until done and lightly brown. Baste several times during cooking process with the sauce.

2 Meanwhile, prepare the sauce. Melt margarine in a large saucepan and add flour. Use wire whisk to make a roux. Add pineapple juice, sherry wine, and vinegar. Bring the sauce to a boil. Check sauce for thickness. Sauce should become a rich brown color and smooth. Serve chicken and sauce on a bed of yellow rice and garnish with a pineapple chunk and parsley (not included in nutritional analysis).

Exchanges
1 1/2 Carbohydrate
2 Lean Meat

Calories 241
   Calories from Fat........... 50
Total Fat .... 6 g
   Saturated Fat................ 1.2 g
   Trans Fat .... 0 g
Cholesterol .... 52 mg
Sodium ....516 mg
Total Carbohydrate ..... 25 g
   Dietary Fiber .... 0 g
   Sugars ....18 g
Protein .... 19 g

Deaconess's Salad

Serves 50 ✦ Serving size: 1 cup

8	medium heads of lettuce
1 1/2	lb tomatoes
3	hardboiled eggs
1 1/2	lb celery
1	lb bell peppers
1	lb capers, drained
1	lb Italian sweet peppers
13	oz fresh anchovies
1	lb green olives, not stuffed, crushed
1	lb ripe olives
2	cups olive oil
1	lb small shrimp, cooked

Chop all ingredients. Cut tomatoes into wedges. Chop eggs into rings for garnish. Mix tomatoes, celery, bell peppers, capers, Italian peppers, anchovies, crushed olives, ripe olives, and olive oil. Save half of this mixture for garnishing the top of the salad. Mix the rest with the chopped lettuce. Layer salad ingredients in a large salad bowl and top with reserved tomato mixture, adding the shrimp and eggs last for garnish. Serve cold.

Exchanges
1 Vegetable
1 Lean Meat
1 1/2 Fat

Calories	149	
Calories from Fat	110	
Total Fat	12	g
Saturated Fat	1.1	g
Trans Fat	0	g
Cholesterol	35	mg
Sodium	487	mg
Total Carbohydrate	5	g
Dietary Fiber	3	g
Sugars	2	g
Protein	5	g

Fresh Mashed Potatoes

Serves 50 ✦ Serving size: 1/4 cup

6	lb fresh potatoes, peeled and quartered
1 1/2	cups nonfat milk
1/2	cup corn-oil stick margarine
2	tsp salt
1	tsp white pepper

In a pot, boil the potato quarters in water for about 30 minutes or until tender. Drain. In a mixing bowl, use a wire whisk to combine the hot potatoes, milk, margarine, salt, and pepper. Mix for 3 minutes at high speed or until smooth.

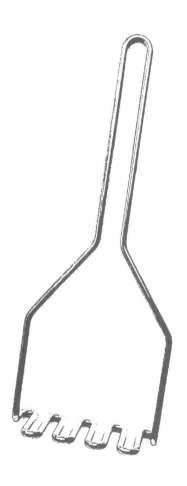

Exchanges
1/2 Starch
1/2 Fat

Calories............................ 55
   Calories from Fat............17
Total Fat .... 2 g
   Saturated Fat............... 0.4 g
   Trans Fat .... 0.3 g
Cholesterol .... 0 mg
Sodium..........................117 mg
Total Carbohydrate .... 9 g
   Dietary Fiber .... 1 g
   Sugars .... 1 g
Protein .... 1 g

Meat Loaf

Serves 50 ✦ Serving size: 1/50 recipe

1 1/2	cups tomato paste
1	cup water
2	cups low-sodium beef stock
1	cup nonfat dry milk
8	lb ground turkey breast
4	eggs
1 1/3	cups onion, chopped
1 3/4	cups celery, chopped
1/4	cup parsley flakes
1	quart + 1 1/2 cups rolled oats
1/2	tsp black pepper
1	Tbsp garlic powder
1	tsp basil
1	tsp oregano
1/2	tsp marjoram
1/2	tsp thyme

Combine tomato paste, water, stock, and dry milk with a mixer. Mix for 2 minutes. Add ground turkey, eggs, onions, celery, oats, and all seasonings. Mix well until blended. Do not overbeat. Form mixture into loaves and place on a cookie sheet. Be sure to smooth the tops of the meat loaf. Bake at 275°F for 1 1/4 hours. Drain fat and let meat loaf sit for 20 minutes. Slice and serve.

Exchanges
1/2 Carbohydrate
2 Lean Meat

Calories	133
Calories from Fat	13
Total Fat	1 g
Saturated Fat	0.4 g
Trans Fat	0 g
Cholesterol	65 mg
Sodium	70 mg
Total Carbohydrate	9 g
Dietary Fiber	1 g
Sugars	1 g
Protein	20 g

Mother of the Church
Meat Sauce with Macaroni

Serves 50 ✦ Serving size: 1/50 recipe

6	lb macaroni
7 1/2	lb 90% lean ground beef
7 1/2	lb ground turkey breast
4	lb onions, chopped
1	lb bell peppers, chopped
3	cloves garlic
2	#10 cans tomatoes (6 lb, 10 oz each)
2	#5 cans tomato juice (46 oz each)
6	Tbsp Worcestershire sauce
	Chili powder to taste
1/4	cup reduced-fat shredded cheese *(optional)*

1 In a large pot of water, cook the macaroni until done.

2 Sauté the beef and turkey together; add onions, peppers, and garlic. Add tomatoes and tomato juice and cook until tomatoes are done. Add Worcestershire sauce and chili powder to taste.

3 Combine the meat mixture with the cooked macaroni. Place into large steam pans. If desired, top the macaroni with a sprinkle of reduced-fat shredded cheese.

Exchanges
2 1/2 Starch
2 Vegetable
3 Lean Meat

Calories 419
    Calories from Fat 64
Total Fat .... 7 g
    Saturated Fat .... 2.5 g
    Trans Fat .... 0.3 g
Cholesterol .... 86 mg
Sodium .... 477 mg
Total Carbohydrate ..... 50 g
    Dietary Fiber .... 4 g
    Sugars .... 9 g
Protein .... 38 g

'Nana Pudding for Everyone

Serves 60 ✦ Serving size: 1/2 cup

- 4 boxes sugar-free banana pudding mix
- 8 cups nonfat milk
- 4 8-oz cartons fat-free whipped topping, thawed
- 20 medium bananas
- 2 cups orange juice
- 4 boxes (12 oz) vanilla wafers

1 Pour sugar-free pudding mix into a medium bowl; mix with the milk. Mix well and set aside in the refrigerator for 5 minutes. Add whipped topping to pudding and refrigerate.

2 In a separate bowl, peel and cut the bananas into small slices. Pour orange juice over the bananas to prevent browning. Drain. In a decorative clear bowl, line the bottom with 1/3 of the vanilla wafers. Cover with pudding, and add a layer of bananas. Repeat layering in this order: vanilla wafers, bananas, and pudding. Leave enough pudding for the remaining top layer. Garnish with extra vanilla wafers. Serve in small martini or wine glasses or small bowls to maintain portion control.

Exchanges
2 1/2 Carbohydrate

Calories	178
Calories from Fat	25
Total Fat	3 g
Saturated Fat	1.2 g
Trans Fat	0 g
Cholesterol	1 mg
Sodium	93 mg
Total Carbohydrate	35 g
Dietary Fiber	2 g
Sugars	19 g
Protein	2 g

Pastor's Dressing

Serves 50 ✦ Serving size: 1/2 cup

1/2 cup canola oil
2 cups chopped celery
1 cup bell pepper, chopped
2 cups chopped onions
1 lb bread crumbs, soft
2 lb dried corn bread stuffing
3 cups low-sodium chicken stock (Use chicken stock on page 216)
Optional spices: sage, poultry seasoning, thyme
(start with 2 Tbsp and increase according to taste)
2 cups egg substitute
1 Tbsp salt
1 Tbsp black pepper

1 In a large saucepan, heat the oil. Add the celery, bell pepper, and onion, and cook until tender. Do not overcook. Remove from stove and put into a mixing bowl.

2 Soak bread crumbs and stuffing in chicken stock from page 216. For your desired degree of moisture, add more stock as needed. If you like it dry, add less stock. After a few minutes, add the bread crumbs and stuffing to the onions, bell pepper, and celery. Add any optional spices. If desired, add turkey giblets (not included in nutritional analysis). Add egg substitute; mix lightly. Add salt and pepper. Pour dressing into an 18 × 20 × 2 1/2-inch baking dish. Bake at 400°F until well browned.

Exchanges
1 1/2 Starch
1/2 Fat

Calories......................... 126
 Calories from Fat........... 30
Total Fat .... 3 g
 Saturated Fat............... 0.2 g
 Trans Fat .... 0 g
Cholesterol .... 0 mg
Sodium..........................414 mg
Total Carbohydrate ..... 20 g
 Dietary Fiber .... 1 g
 Sugars .... 2 g
Protein .... 4 g

Pastor's Oven-Baked Chicken

Serves 50 ✦ Serving size: 1/50 recipe

24	lb chicken, cut into pieces, skin removed
3 1/2	cups all-purpose flour
3 1/4	cups nonfat dry milk
1 1/2	Tbsp poultry seasoning
1	Tbsp black pepper
1 1/2	tsp paprika
2	Tbsp garlic powder
	Nonstick cooking spray

Rinse chicken in cold water; drain well. Combine flour, dry milk, poultry seasoning, pepper, paprika, and garlic powder. Mix well. Spray chicken with nonstick cooking spray and toss in flour mixture. Place chicken pieces on a greased cookie sheet. Bake at 350°F for 35 minutes, until golden brown. If a crispier chicken is desired, bake at 400°F, but be careful not to burn.

Exchanges
1/2 Starch
3 Very Lean Meat
1 Fat

Calories	183	
Calories from Fat	48	
Total Fat	5	g
Saturated Fat	1.4	g
Trans Fat	0	g
Cholesterol	63	mg
Sodium	85	mg
Total Carbohydrate	9	g
Dietary Fiber	0	g
Sugars	3	g
Protein	23	g

Sistah Addie Mae's Stew Beef

Serves 50 ✦ Serving size: 1/50 recipe

1	lb flour
18	lb lean stew beef cuts
1	lb onions, chopped
2 3/4	gallons low-sodium beef stock (Use beef stock on page 216)
6	lb carrots
6	lb potatoes, diced or whole
1	#10 can crushed tomatoes (6 lb, 10 oz)
2	Tbsp salt
2	Tbsp black pepper
1	#10 can cooked onions (6 lb, 10 oz)
1	lb cooked green peas

Rub the flour into the meat. Divide the meat among two roasting pans, sprinkle with onions, and braise at 350°F, until meat is half done (about 30 minutes). Put the meat into one large pan. Add the beef stock (use the recipe on page 216) and the carrots. Cook for 20 minutes. Add the diced or whole new potatoes. Cook for 15 minutes. Add the tomatoes and continue cooking until meat and vegetables are done and tender. Add salt and pepper. Remove from oven and add the #10 can of cooked onions. Pan up the stew and sprinkle with green peas.

Exchanges
1 1/2 Starch
2 Vegetables
3 Lean Meat

Calories........................ 306
   Calories from Fat........... 62
Total Fat .... 7 g
   Saturated Fat................2.1 g
   Trans Fat .... 0 g
Cholesterol .... 85 mg
Sodium........................714 mg
Total Carbohydrate ..... 30 g
   Dietary Fiber .... 5 g
   Sugars .... 7 g
Protein ....31 g

Sistah Mabel's Macaroni and Cheese

Serves 50 ✦ Serving size: 1/50 recipe

2	lb elbow macaroni
3/4	lb light, soft, tub margarine
3/4	lb all-purpose flour
2	tsp salt
1	Tbsp dry mustard
1	Tbsp white pepper
1	Tbsp paprika
5	quarts nonfat milk
2	tsp Worcestershire sauce
3/4	lb reduced-fat cheddar cheese, shredded
1 3/4	lb fat-free cheddar cheese
1/2	cup freshly grated Parmesan cheese

Cook macaroni in boiling water until firm and tender. Drain and rinse in cold water. Melt the margarine in a stock pot. Combine flour, salt, dry mustard, white pepper, and paprika in a bowl. Add to melted margarine and cook for 2 minutes over medium heat, stirring continuously. Do not brown. Slowly add the milk to the flour mixture, stirring constantly, until smooth and thickened. Add Worcestershire sauce and cheeses to sauce until cheese melts. Combine well-drained macaroni and sauce. Mix well; bake uncovered at 325°F for 25 minutes until lightly browned.

Exchanges
1 1/2 Starch
1 Lean Meat

Calories	191	
Calories from Fat	40	
Total Fat	4	g
Saturated Fat	1.4	g
Trans Fat	0	g
Cholesterol	9	mg
Sodium	414	mg
Total Carbohydrate	24	g
Dietary Fiber	1	g
Sugars	6	g
Protein	13	g

Soul Sistah Slaw

Serves 50 ✦ Serving size: 1/2 cup

9	lb shredded cabbage
1 1/8	cups Splenda® Sugar Blend for Baking
1 1/2	cups bell pepper, thinly chopped
1 1/2	cups grated carrots
1/2	cup grated onion
1/4	cup vinegar, as desired
3 1/4	cups reduced-fat mayonnaise
	Salt-free seasoning, as desired *(optional)*
1	12-oz can evaporated skim milk

Chop the cabbage in a food processor. In a large mixing bowl, combine cabbage with Splenda®, bell pepper, carrots, and onions. Add the vinegar and mayonnaise. If desired, add salt-free seasoning. Toss gently. Add milk and mix well.

Exchanges
1/2 Carbohydrate
1 Vegetable
1 Fat

Calories.........................102
   Calories from Fat............51
Total Fat .... 6 g
   Saturated Fat............... 0.9 g
   Trans Fat .... 0 g
Cholesterol .... 5 mg
Sodium.........................170 mg
Total Carbohydrate ..... 12 g
   Dietary Fiber .... 2 g
   Sugars .... 9 g
Protein .... 2 g

Teriyaki Chicken

50 servings ✦ Serving size: 1 thigh

1	cup lemon juice
3/4	cup lite soy sauce
2/3	cup canola oil
1/2	cup catsup
1/2	tsp black pepper
1/2	tsp garlic powder
12	lb skinless chicken thighs

1 In a bowl, whisk together the lemon juice, soy sauce, canola oil, catsup, pepper, and garlic powder until smooth. Set aside.

2 Place 50 chicken pieces on a lightly greased baking sheet and pour 1 cup of sauce over each piece. Bake at 325°F for 60 minutes, until golden brown. Place in a serving pan and pour remaining sauce over the chicken. Serve hot.

Exchanges
2 Lean Meat
1/2 Fat

Calories	142	
Calories from Fat	79	
Total Fat	9	g
Saturated Fat	1.8	g
Trans Fat	0	g
Cholesterol	50	mg
Sodium	213	mg
Total Carbohydrate	1	g
Dietary Fiber	0	g
Sugars	1	g
Protein	14	g

Soul Food
Index

Alphabetical list of recipes

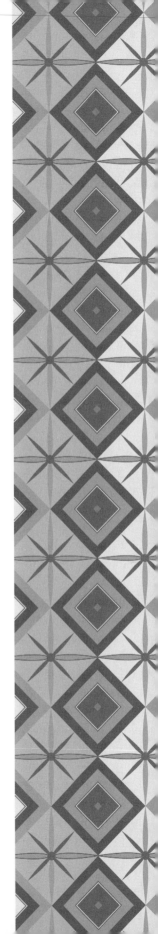

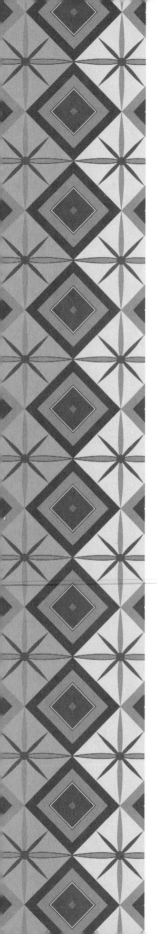

Subject list of recipes